THE
SCALABLE
PRACTICE

The Missing Role
to Grow Your Practice
Faster & Easier

Luke Infinger

The Scalable Practice

ISBN-13: 978-1-990476-08-2

Published by: Expert Author Press
https://www.expertauthorpress.com/

Canadian Address:
1908 – 1251 Cardero Street,
Vancouver, BC, Canada, V6G 2H9
Phone: (604) 941-3041
info@expertauthorpress.com

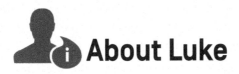 # About Luke

Back in May 2012, right after I graduated from the Savannah College of Art and Design (SCAD) with a degree in motion graphics, I targeted a very niched motion graphics and design shop in New York City for a job. I sent everyone in the company LinkedIn messages until a guy, who was also a SCAD grad, got me in for an interview. The boss offered me an internship, but I countered, asking for a full-time role, telling him I had another offer. I promised that if he gave me a shot, I'd give it everything. After he hired me, he told the team at a company retreat, "Luke knew exactly what he wanted and went for it."

I chose the company because I had seen the high-quality work they were doing and wanted to be a part of that. They did the promos for big shows, and their brand attracted me. Unfortunately, when I got there, the culture sucked. It was a sweatshop. We worked from 10 a.m. to midnight, had to take our hard drives home to keep working on projects over the weekend, and the boss yelled at people almost every day. I made less money than it took to live in the city, but for the year I was there, I crushed it. I did the entire season three promos for Game of Thrones with one other guy's help.

My biggest takeaway from that experience was to treat people the way you want to be treated. It doesn't mean you have to be soft, but simply be caring, fair, and honest and do what's best for others. You need to be wildly passionate about your role and still maintain a healthy work-life balance. As an employer, you need to believe in that, and you need to hire people who think similarly. What I also learned from that experience, however, is that things can always be worse. In fact, most people who complain about their jobs sometimes don't understand how good they have it.

After I left, Justin Hual and I started HIP, a company specializing in orthodontic marketing and growth strategies. Since then, it's been a phenomenal ride with amazing orthodontists and dentists, and I have not looked back. We built the company from the ground up, and it's based on our core values of Hunger, Integrity, and Passion (HIP). You will find them reflected through every process in our business and every interaction with our team.

Table of Contents

Introduction

Why the Scalable Practice?

In February 2016, I had my first meeting with Dr. Ben Fishbein. At that time, Fishbein Orthodontics had about 20 team members, three locations (two were small satellites), and one doctor. They produced around 2 million dollars.

Long story short, we began working together soon after. Initially, they brought us in to deliver some photos and videos, and we ran an Invisalign campaign. We began to earn their trust and became their digital marketing partners. Essentially, we started to oversee and deliver their digital ads (Facebook, Instagram, Google), SEO, and Reputation Management. We began to hone in on the process of tracking leads moving through the patient journey and starting treatment.

With Fishbein, I will be honest: It was fairly easy. We were spoiled!

They had their processes down. They tracked everything. They had an amazing mindset and a bulletproof scheduling process. We instantly knew it was working.

As we continued to work and meet with them to discuss strategies, I quickly noticed that Dr. Fishbein wasn't the one managing everything and calling all the shots; he had empowered a leadership team early on. The two main people I started reporting to at the time were Amanda Floyd (COO) and Aliza Ray (Director of Marketing).

Dr. Ben trusted his team to own their roles and be accountable for their projects, tasks, successes, and failures. Because of that, the business began to grow like wildfire.

There are four main components of any business:

1. Marketing
2. Sales
3. Operations
4. Finance

It appeared that Dr. Fishbein knew this very early in the game and made a strategic plan for each of them that would ultimately remove him from having to spend a lot of time—and in most cases, zero time—in each quadrant of the business.

He was now free to see a lot of patients and figure out how to do it efficiently.

If you are business savvy, you probably think, *Luke, this is obvious: the owner and visionary can't do it all.* Think of Apple, Starbucks, or any successful company, for that matter. Each has an amazing team in place to facilitate growth.

However, we typically only hear about the growers. When

was the last time a failing small business was in the spotlight?

Yet, 20% of new businesses fail in the first two years, 45% in the first five years, and 65% in the first ten years. There is just as much, if not more, to learn from the failing businesses as there is from the growing businesses.

I will go ahead and say it: Orthodontists typically aren't super business savvy. I do not mean this as an insult. They were not trained to run a business. Yet, here you are, reading this book, educating yourself, and hopefully, being able to get at least 1% better (though I hope it is much more than that!) and moving forward to new heights.

My mission in starting HIP and choosing to be the best we can be is to help orthodontists make the best decisions with their time, money, marketing, and health. (I added health about 2 years ago as it became a huge part of my life due to a journey I had to go through myself).

We often hear, "It's easier said than done." That's because we love our comfort zones. As much as we hate to admit it, most humans don't like change. We are creatures of habit.

If you are aware of this, you can fight it. You can change quickly. The mind is amazing, and God gave us the ability to do the unimaginable.

Who would have thought the fastest-growing orthodontist would be in Pensacola, Florida? It's a small Navy town with a super-chill beach vibe.

But it happened!

This book is designed to break down the key business role inside the practice and show you how to turn your practice into a rocket ship. Suppose this isn't what you want, and you want to keep your team small, stay under 3 million in production, take more days off, and bring in associates with somewhat low revenue (I recommend it around 4 to 6 million in production depending on multiple variables).

In that case, you may want to:

1. Send this book back to me.
2. Use it as a fire starter.
3. Give it to a friend or peer who wants to blow the doors off their practice.

I was once told, "Hire for what you can't do, not what you can do."

I've met many orthodontists who bring in associates (who can do what they do) way too soon just so they can take more days off or be the visionary—or, even worse, manager—of their practice. Then, they say, "But I am not taking home enough, and we can't grow." (I am not knocking being a visionary; I will break this down in the first chapter. My point is that, in some cases, it's an excuse to check out and not be stressed or worried about the responsibility of seeing more patients).

Instead, they should be hiring business people to handle anything and everything outside of the clinic and treating patients. Once that is in place and you are experiencing rapid growth, THEN look to bring in associates.

This will maintain healthy margins and allow you to take home a more than fair owner's salary and distribution. In addition, you'll be able to pay competitive salaries and bonus positions better than 99% of other practices.

If this is what you want, keep reading, make a plan with a timeline to implement, set your goals, and reach out to me with any questions. I am here to help with no strings attached.

Onward and upward!

Luke Infinger, Co-Founder & CEO at HIP

CHAPTER
Becoming the Visionary

Becoming an orthodontist is a big deal. It's expensive, an exceptional amount of work, and few people can do it. It's also very lucrative. Opening a practice or working in another office can make you more money than most people can ever dream of making. For all your hard work, it's truly a blessing, but it can also be a trap that I have seen many doctors fall into. You see, just opening your doors and hanging out your shingle can be enough for your practice to produce one to 1.2 million per year. Well, maybe it's not that easy, but it's not a bad gig, right? But considering that you graduate with about 600-800 thousand dollars of debt, rising costs, and increased competition, it can also be a bit daunting.

Now you can attend some practice management courses and get some help running your practice and push that number up a bit. The fact is, most orthodontists I come across want more new patients so they can increase production. Why? Well, most likely, their operating costs, practice ambitions, and lifestyle are at odds, and they feel the need to generate more income to bring things into balance. Simply put, their back is up against the wall. When I go to orthodontic seminars and conferences, doctors are always telling each other about things they have done to grow their practices. It seems like everyone is looking for that magic bullet that brings all the patients they need through their doors.

But what's it all for? I've talked to hundreds of orthodontists, visited their practices, and worked with many of them. Across the board, the most common thing I hear is, "Luke, we just need more patients." That's fine, and I can help them get those patients. Still, they always discover that there is much more involved in increasing production than simply hiring a marketing company, opening a new location, or advertising low fees. Just because another doctor at a seminar did that one thing and doubled their practice does not mean that you can do the same thing and expect a similar result.

To be sustainable, any growth changes you make require two foundational factors in your practice:

1. You absolutely must have your processes and systems nailed down.
2. The right team members have to OWN specific roles and hold everyone accountable and be aligned with your mission and vision.

Without these two critical elements in place, changes

will fall to pieces quickly, the team will get frustrated, and everyone learns that if they wait it out, your great new idea will fall through the cracks. Ultimately, the debt keeps piling up, and you will not grow to where you really want to be.

If this sounds all too familiar, don't worry. The good news is it's not that hard to create the foundation that great practices are built on if you know your goals and have a great mindset. You just need to choose the practice model you want, take baby steps daily, and invest in the right people.

So, what exactly is holding people back from increasing their production, then? The main reason is this: they don't have a clear vision for their practice and life. Without the definite direction laid out by that vision, all their staff, operations, processes, and goals lack a target to be measured against. The doctor is left watching things break down or blow up as they plod along putting out fires, trying to maintain the status quo. They operate in constant, low-grade frustration, trying to keep up with their lifestyle and contemplating the secret to making a practice work.

If you have read Books #1 and #2 of our Orthodontic Practice Growth Series, you will have discovered many practical ideas, procedures, and scripts that will help you get more new patients and increase production. We showed you how the fastest-growing practices in the nation train their front desks and scheduling teams to turn more leads into prospective patients. We looked inside some of their offices to see how their treatment coordinators sell their services to prospective patients and turn over 80% of them into happy and satisfied, same-day starts. If you and your team have studied those two books, you have all the tips, tricks, strategies, processes, and procedures to make it happen. It's simply a matter of implementation. Your operations must be top-notch, and the patient experience has to be second to none. Are you and your team committed to doing what it takes by training, practicing, and roleplaying to get your operations online and humming like the top 1% orthodontic offices?

Are You Cut Out for Scalable Growth?

If you have started paying more attention to the things that you would like to change or upgrade in your office, and you are serious about getting your whole team on board, you may be ready to take the leap and join the peak performers in your profession. You've seen their active social media accounts, thoughtfully-designed websites, perfectly curated offices, and wonderfully creative staff delivering exceptional service. You can find them everywhere in their community, doing outreach, providing sponsorships, and running compelling ads. Their multiple locations pop up throughout the state, and all seem to thrive. If you have the want and desire to grow to that level, it's time to ask yourself whether or not you are cut out for scalable growth.

As a growth partner with different practices in this industry, I've gotten to know enough orthodontists to understand that it can happen for those with the right mindset. What you must understand is that these doctors are a special breed. They don't think like the average orthodontist. They see their practice as a business whose purpose is to provide excellent service to as many people in the community as possible. They are the CEO and visionary of their practice and not just an orthodontist. It's all about the business and the size of the impact they can make as it grows. It's not about them and what they can get out of it. All the rewards that you see them reap are side effects of their massive desire to serve. It's what they value, and it's coded in their DNA.

It's time to ask yourself some serious questions. Why do you want to grow? If you have a number in mind, why have you chosen that number? What happens when you hit that number? Will you settle down and be comfortable with maintaining your practice at that level, or will you celebrate the achievement and set the next target? Your answers to these questions will determine if you are part of that special breed or if you are a different type of orthodontist. There are no right or wrong answers, and if you don't want what the industry's top performers want, that's perfectly okay and noble. It is very important to know how you want to use the information in this book, if indeed you want to use it at all.

Some doctors are comfortable growing to the point that supports their desired lifestyle. Maybe you just want a well-run, profitable, and sustainable business that allows you to do five million in production and take home two. Perhaps you don't even want the perceived hassle of managing all the people necessary to grow to that level and are happy with a tight ship that you can count on to give you a take-home of $800,000. All these desires and objectives are fine. It's just very important to know what you want and why. Your dreams are your own, and no one can judge you for them.

If you answer the questions above and discover that you want to make enough money to spend time with your family and friends, take lots of great vacations, build your dream home, drive nice cars, or anything else you can imagine, that's great! Your "why" is about providing a lifestyle for yourself and making the money it takes to do so. We must all take care of our own needs first so we can be of service to others. But if your answers reveal that you want to be of greater service to others and that you want to grow your reach as large as possible to have the biggest influence possible on your community, then your "why" is about serving others. It's not about you.

I know there are many more components to your "why" than this, but the distinction between whether it is about you or others is critical in developing the vision for your practice.

Lifestyle vs. Scaleable Practice

Regardless of the practice you plan to build, you should see yourself as the CEO and visionary for your business. How big you want to grow will determine whether you want to move beyond this chapter or simply work through the processes in this chapter and focus on the first two books in the Orthodontic Practice Growth Series. If you are happy with running a tight ship that lets you take home a high six-figure to seven-figure salary, depending on your margins, you may not need to read on. If you want to grow past the three million mark into the medium practice size range, you may want to consider implementing what I have to share in this book. If your goal is to keep growing and setting new goals as you reach them, this book is definitely for you.

Think about the type of practice you want. Are you building a lifestyle practice where your people are highly trained in the operation of the business, so you just need to show up, do what you do best, then leave to dedicate your time and energy to other things in your life? Do you have your sights set on a scalable practice that you plan on doubling, tripling, or even quadrupling? Do you see yourself with multiple locations and teams that know how to run them so they all reflect your values and brand? Both practices require a vision and a significant amount of time, energy, and dedication to create them. The difference is that the lifestyle practice has a target that, once reached, is maintained because the goal has been achieved. The scalable practice is all about increasing growth to maximize impact. When a goal is achieved, the visionary is already looking at the next level they can shoot for. For either practice, you must have a clear vision to reach your goal.

What's Your Vision?

Think a little deeper. As you and your team work to build your practice, who is involved in that journey? What brand do you want your patients and community to buy into? What culture do you need in your practice to uphold that brand? How do you want your patients to feel? Who will take the reigns and ensure the vision becomes a reality?

If your answer to the last question is "me," I urge you to think about where your time is best spent. An orthodontist is making the most money when they are chairside seeing patients. Executing the vision is a full-time job and must be given to someone qualified to do it. You certainly did not spend ten-plus years studying to be in management, but some people did go to school for this and have the experience to put the systems in place to make the vision come to life.

As you answer those questions, what words or phrases come to mind? When you think about your practice, how would you describe it? If you had your ideal practice, what would the Google reviews say? How would your patients talk about your practice to their friends? This is a great way to discover the words or phrases for your core values.

Your Core Values Bring Your Vision to Life

Your core values define your culture and who you are as a person. Everything you do in your business must revolve around those core values. It's showcased in all your employee processes, including hiring, firing, reviews, and recognition. They are the consistent messaging in every team meeting, every patient interaction, and every procedure that takes place within your office. Without them, your practice would lack meaning, significance, heart, and clarity. Without them, there's no way to grow.

Dr. Farina, CEO of Farina Orthodontics, has his core values in his entryway for his team and patients to see every time they come into the office. This vibrant and colorful display takes up a huge chunk of the wall, outlining the true values he believes make up the entire existence of his practice:

1. Deliver WOW Through Service & Smiles.

2. Promising High Energy and High Fives.

3. Creating an Environment Where We Think Big, Have Fun, and Do Good.

4. Fostering a Culture of Warmth and Belonging Where Everyone is Welcome.

5. Make It Simple. Get It Done.

6. Be Present, Clear, and Humble.

7. One Team. One Family. One Vision.

8. Encourage and Embrace Change.

9. Choosing Passion and Commitment Over Convenience.

10. It's Up to Me to Make It Be.

Dr. Farina's decision to broadcast his core values in a bold and well-designed way on his wall is a strategic one. He knows the only way to make his vision come to life is by sharing his core values with his team and patients. If you don't tell people what your core values are, how will you attract like-minded people who want to promote the same values? If your people don't buy into those values, they are doing your practice a disservice. Dr. Farina cultivated a team that stands behind every single core value listed above. Over the last three years, we've seen him double his practice and continue to make great strides with his team toward his next goal.

Take the time to develop a list of core values and share them with your team. They may have differing views on them initially, but I encourage you to work with your team to form what you believe to be the backbone and heart of your practice.

Code Your Biggest Values in Your DNA

When you think of massive companies like the Ritz Carlton, Starbucks, and Chick-fil-A, what's the first thing that comes to mind? Probably excellent customer service because that's what keeps us going back. When there's a level of consistency a company brings to the public sphere that is unmatched by competitors, you can't help but feel that it's embedded in their DNA. That level of attention and consistency did not happen by accident. That is because their CEO had a vision from the get-go and made it happen from day one. You cannot be the only person who makes up your company's DNA—it must be shared by 100% of your company. It's the one thing that makes you different from your competitors. When you decide what your DNA is, the rest of your core values align to support it. Your DNA is the bedrock of your success. Everything else is built upon it.

Effective communication and excellent service: those two factors make up the DNA of my company, HIP. It's what I put out to the world and what I want them to think of when they think about the services my company provides. And if you're doing it the right way, you should be hearing it: whether that's verbally by your patients or written in reviews.

I went through the Google reviews on HIP's website to see if that messaging is reflected in our customer responses:

"Impossibly responsive."

"Live on their phones and laptops—Can call anytime if I need anything."

"They made the transition painless."

"Luke and his team go out of their way to give value and quality of service."

"Super professional and prompt."

"Extremely responsive."

The vision, core values, and DNA of your practice should be so well-defined and reflected in your processes that your patients start to state it back to you. This is the standard that you want to have your vision crafted to. If you accomplish this and your whole team buys in and reflects it in every patient interaction, it will come to be.

Developing Your Growth Plan : From Your Core Values to Your Future Goals

With the right mindset to get you there, you can achieve all the goals you set for yourself and your practice. But like all things in life, it won't come to you overnight. There is a significant amount of reflecting, planning, organizing, and executing that will have to take place to get you there—not just by you but by your entire team. Everyone involved in this process has to get on board for your vision to come to life. And that process can be quite daunting and scary, and it's hard to know where to start. It starts with a vision, some core values, a strong DNA, and the right people in the right seats to take you there. You will also need to have the right operations in place and the right people managing all of the moving parts that your practice requires to grow successfully.

That means everyone needs to focus on one target at the same time.

To help you do this, you need an operating system. One that I particularly like and worked for me is the Entrepreneurial Operating System (EOS), eosworldwide. com. It's a set of simple concepts and practical tools that will help you plan and execute the vision you have for your practice. Their concepts have inspired HIP to develop our own template for tracking visions and goals, which I call the Orthodontic Practice Operating System.

Scan this QR code to download it—It's the first step to starting your journey.

The Orthodontic Practice Operating System will enable you to get that vision out of your head and onto paper, aiding you and your team to efficiently go through the motions of making your ideal practice a reality.

It includes a series of questions you will need to answer thoughtfully to help fill in the gaps about what your plan is for growth. These questions include:

1. What are your core values?
2. What is the bedrock of your success (DNA)?
3. What is your core focus?
4. What is your 10-year target?

5. What are your 3 uniques?

6. What is your proven process?

7. What is your guarantee?

8. What is your marketing strategy?

9. Who is your target market?

10. What is your 3-year picture?

11. What is your 1-year plan?

12. What are your quarterly rocks?

13. What are your issues and/or liabilities?

To help get you started, I've included an example of the Orthodontic Practice Operating System that outlines all of the factors involved in a 10-year plan.

Also, here is a suggested meeting schedule to ensure you and your team stay on track and continually review the practice's progress. Use the Orthodontic Practice Operating System to help drive the meeting agendas.

As you can see, it is specific, measurable, and realistic. It is our mission, vision, core values, DNA, short-term goals, long-term goals, the obstacles standing in our way, and our priorities to take those obstacles down. It is thoughtful, well-executed, and agreed upon by the entire HIP leadership team.

Dr. Connor Despot, CEO of SmileCrew Orthodontics, knows the importance of utilizing an operating system to successfully grow his business:

> *"To get anywhere, you have to have goals. Like that old saying, "Failure to plan is planning to fail." If you don't set goals, you have no way to figure out or assess where you're at. But beyond that, you need an operating system. Most orthodontists don't know much about business, but you need a way to operate. EOS helps everyone stay aligned, and it creates a huge level of accountability and levels of oversight. People can see where they're doing well and where they're not doing well. There are metrics and measurable things that we look at."*

He continues:

> *"If you don't have an operating system, it's very tough for one or two people to handle. It becomes too much. You have to have levels of accountability. And you have to have people that are accountable for people, and those people are accountable for people. You should have an accountability chart that needs to be published to your whole organization, so everyone knows where they stand on that accountability chart, their roles, whom they answer to, who their boss is, and so on."*

Like the many businesses that have thrived by using EOS templates to track their vision and goals, Dr. Despot has an idea of where he wants to be in 10 years:

> *"My goal is to get to eight offices by 2031. We want to provide 20,000 confident, attractive, healthy smiles. We want to be able to donate 500 smiles to the community.*

We want to give back to the families in our community that need orthodontic treatment but can't afford it. For example, we have a patient who lost his mom right after he started treatment. Well, that treatment is now free for that kid. When those things happen, treatment becomes free for those kids. That's a smile that's donated, and it's a way we give back to those families who have already gone through enough. We also want to give $200,000 back to the community, whether that's through school sponsorships or scholarships, or things like that."

Teamwork Makes the Dream Work

You have a team in place for a reason. They're there to bring your vision to life. It's easy to have all of these goals if your team believes in you and your vision. You can't do this alone, and the more you come to terms with that, the better off you'll be.

I encourage you to start making active changes and relinquish your control of practice operations to someone else who is better equipped to execute your vision. Your practice may or may not be in a position to take this step now, but I want you to start planning for it. As the orthodontist, you need to be the CEO, visionary, and technician who is chairside seeing patients. Doing anything else is losing money.

Please don't take the word technician the wrong way. It comes from the book, The E-Myth Revisited: Why Most Small Businesses Don't Work and What to Do About It by Michael Gerber. It's about professionals and people with specialized skills who have never studied business or operated a company. When they decide it would be wonderful to have their own shop, company, or practice, they have what he calls "the entrepreneurial seizure." He says that for this person to succeed, they need to wear three hats, or they will end up overworked, frustrated, and tormented by the craziest boss they've ever had: themselves. Instead, he encourages new business owners to wear the technician hat and focus on doing what they're trained in. But at the same time, wear the other two hats—the entrepreneur hat and the manager hat—to develop their business in the very beginning.

As your practice grows, you want to move out of management altogether and leave it to the person responsible for implementing your ideas into systems to make the business sustainable. You can't do everything forever if you want your business to grow!

So, who is this person? The next chapter introduces the crucial person who will take your vision by the horns and break it into targets and milestones. This person will free you to do what you do best while they integrate your vision into the operations of your practice. This person is your Chief Operating Officer (COO), and if your practice is crossing the line from small to medium-sized (breaking the three million mark), it's time to consider hiring one. If you're curious to know who this person is and what they do, read on. The next chapter is dedicated to them, and the rest of the book is their domain.

Implementing the Integrator

Let's face the facts: Running a multimillion-dollar company is a full-time job, as is being a busy and successful orthodontist. You can't do both. Since you made it here, past the first chapter and all its warnings, I assume you want to build your practice like a scalable business. From this point forward, we will be discussing all aspects of the operations of an orthodontic practice and how the Chief Operating Officer (COO), or the integrator of your vision, pulls them all together and aligns them with your core values and DNA.

When you work through the Operating System in the previous chapter, you will understand that the growth you want to achieve for your practice is not something that will simply manifest by hoping it will come to you. It needs to be thoroughly planned and executed with your team. You'll have to set quarterly priorities, understand the key obstacles interfering with those priorities, and learn how to overcome them. You'll have to set targets to work towards in your one-year mark, your three-year mark, and even your ten-year mark if you're feeling ambitious.

This is way too much for one person to do on their own. You'll need a leadership team who believes in your vision and is willing to work hard to make it a reality. The head of that leadership team is your COO. The COO is your integrator who will believe in your vision and integrate it into your practice.

Who Should Be Your COO?

What should this person look like? What qualities should they have? Why is it necessary to hire one? If you're the brain behind the practice, then they're the hands. You think and come up with ideas, and they take action on them. They should be able to lead a team to excellence and work with honesty, integrity, and drive. The COO is working both behind the scenes and on the front deck, problem-solving, organizing, and communicating with your leadership team to relay your core values.

They are accountable for the growth of your practice. If they can't get your message across efficiently, then they're in the wrong seat. Just like you went to dental school and completed your orthodontic residency to specialize as an orthodontist, they've specialized in operations and business, whether through business programs or learning hands-on in previous organizations.

Without them, substantial growth would be near impossible to achieve.

They have pretty big shoes to fill by joining your team. It's not an easy job to bring someone's vision to life. So, when you hire a COO, they shouldn't be thought of as just another employee. They should be thought of as your business partner. That means when you have ideas, they need to know about them. You may come up with ten ideas every day, and your COO needs to be honest and transparent with you about which ideas full-on suck and which ones can be brought to life.

The Predictive Index: The Attributes of the Ideal COO

To give you an idea of the attributes you should be looking for in your ideal COO, I've included the Predictive Index (PI) report of my own COO, HIP's very own Justin Hual. Justin is considered a Strategist, according to PI, known for his sense of urgency and ability to drive results. You can scan this QR code to view his full report.

Strongest Behaviors

Justin will most strongly express the following behaviors:

- Proactivity, assertiveness, and a sense of urgency in driving to reach personal goals. Openly challenges the world.

- Independent in putting forth their own ideas, which are often innovative and, if implemented, cause change. Resourcefully works through or around anything blocking completion of what they want to accomplish; aggressive when challenged.

- Impatient for results, puts pressure on themself and others for rapid implementation, and is far less productive when doing routine work.

- Task-focused; quickly notices and pushes to fix technical problems, assertively cutting through any personal and emotional issues. Has aptitude to spot trends in data or figure out how complex systems work.

- Independent, analytical, critical; a creative thinker and action-oriented; little need for external validation before action. Private.

- Authoritative and direct, driven to accomplish personal goals; push through roadblocks assertively. Communication is direct, to the point, and sometimes brusque.

- Careful with rules; precise, "by the book," fast-paced, and literal in interpreting rules, schedules, and results.

- Detail-oriented and thorough; works to ensure things don't fall through the cracks and follow up to ensure they're done properly and on time.

- Driven to achieve operational efficiencies: thinks about what needs to be done and how it can be done as fast as possible while maintaining a high-quality outcome. Impatient with routines.

Summary

Justin is an intense, results-oriented self-starter whose drive and sense of urgency are tempered and disciplined by a concern for the accuracy and quality of the work. His approach to activities and responsibilities will be well-thought-out, based on thorough analysis and detailed knowledge of all pertinent facts.

Strongly technically oriented, he has confidence in his own professional knowledge and ability to get things done quickly and correctly. With experience, he will develop a high level of expertise and be very aware of mistakes committed by himself or others. Justin takes work and responsibilities seriously and expects others to do the same.

In social matters, he is reserved and private, with little interest in "small talk." Interest and energy will be focused primarily on the work, and in general, he is more comfortable and open in the work environment than in purely social situations. In the work environment, they are factual, direct, and authoritative.

Imaginative and venturesome, he is creative and capable of developing new ideas, systems, plans, or technology, or of analyzing and improving old ones. They rely primarily on their own knowledge and thinking, with little reference to others, to get things done. Justin sets a high, exacting personal standard and generally finds that others do not meet it. To earn trust, someone must consistently meet that standard and get results. If someone can do that, Justin will do what's needed to work with them whenever collaboration is needed.

He may be perceived by others as aloof but will earn respect for their knowledge, work, and the soundness of the decisions that they make.

Management Strategies

To maximize effectiveness, productivity, and job satisfaction, consider providing Justin with the following:

- Opportunities to broaden technical knowledge and gain experience in increasingly responsible positions.
- As much autonomy as possible in setting priorities, expressing ideas, and putting them into action.

- Recognition for tangible results obtained, rather than for political or selling skills.

- Freedom from repetition.

- Technical challenges that require innovative solutions.

HIP wouldn't be where it currently stands without his contribution. He continuously sees HIP's vision through and does whatever he can in his power to make our dreams a reality. If you want to learn more about the Strategist personality type and dive deep into the profile, please scan this QR code.

Promoting Internally or Hiring Externally: Which Path Is Right?

Many businesses need help deciding whether to promote within their own organization or hire externally to fill roles. You want to ensure you're putting the right people in the right seats, but it's sometimes hard to fully gauge what the right decision is.

Promoting Internally

If you already have someone in your office that comes to mind when you think of your future COO, then that's great! It wouldn't make sense to grow your practice without giving them the chance to grow with you. If Jennifer from your sales team has the perfect mindset, abilities, and capacity to be your right-hand woman, give her that opportunity to show you that she's more than capable of getting the job done.

However, I would advise that before you make this decision, you should ensure that the person you are promoting internally is as well-versed and knowledgeable in ALL areas of your practice as possible. This means they should have experience in every department and understand the fundamental responsibilities of every role within those departments. Because if they can't understand it, then how will they be able to manage it? The COO is responsible for overseeing all of the day-to-day operations of your business. If they're required to lead and manage all of your department directors and managers, they have a lot more credibility if they understand the role because they have done it.

Janet Moser, COO of AllSmiles Orthodontics, started as a treatment coordinator and was promoted to team leader (office manager) years before she became the COO of an eight-figure practice. Janet understands the necessity of learning each role and department before moving up, so she instills the same process in all of her new hires:

> *"I give a lot of credit to Dr. McDowell for putting his faith and trust in me and giving me the autonomy, tools, and coaching to be successful in this role. But I think working my way up to this position has worked in my favor because I've earned the respect of my team. They've seen me get my hands dirty over the years and put in the work. And when they need help, I'm more than willing*

to help them. If they don't see me being a team player, how can I expect them to be? My number one thing is to lead by example. That's why I honestly believe that when you first get hired here, you have to learn everything. You have to have a chance to be trained in all of the different roles, and then we find the best one that works for you and your skills. You'll do that role on the day-to-day, but if we're down a person or a department needs another set of hands, you'll easily jump right in. Specialized roles, but knowledgeable in everything."

Hiring Externally

If you don't have a rockstar treatment coordinator turned COO like Janet to promote within your practice currently, then that's also fine. There are multiple job boards you can use and also agencies you can hire to help you with the recruitment process. Wiseman Strategies, for example, helps companies find their ideal talent by aiding with the entire recruitment process. They'll help you get the right people in the right seats, source the right candidates, prepare for the interview, and create a great interview experience (We'll go into more detail on Wiseman Strategies in Chapter 5).

But before jumping to put that ad on Indeed or Workopolis, you need to make sure your COO job description is fully tailored to the role and includes ALL of the core values so that you can find someone who believes in them.

Here are some of the main duties and responsibilities

you should expect your COO to do as the operational leader of your practice:

- Oversee the daily operations of the practice and drive results from both an operational and financial perspective while working closely with the CEO and other leadership team members.

- Measure actual budgetary performance (revenue, expense, staffing) against standards and ensures variances are within established targets.

- Develop and implement operational processes, protocols, policies, and procedures on efficiency and scalability.

- Create an environment that facilitates innovative delivery of care for the community it serves.

- Establish mechanisms to encourage innovation and incorporate best-practice findings into standards of practice and policies and procedures.

- Maintain familiarity with the operational procedures at all levels of the organization.

- Empower all teams with the autonomy and resources they need to complete initiatives.

- Partner with the leadership team to accomplish short and long-term operational goals.

- Set challenging but realistic goals for growth, performance, and profitability.

- Identify potential areas of geographic expansion through organic growth or acquisition.

- Analyze and interpret data and metrics.

- Measure and report on operational performance and develops plans to improve relevant key performance indicators (KPIs).

- Provide management to staff and guidance in alignment with the business plan and strategic vision.

- Lead employees by example to reinforce a culture of excellence and establish policies that promote company culture and vision.

- Maintain positive, productive relationships with partners, vendors, and affiliates.

- Always represent the company positively through a success-oriented and professional demeanor.

Scan this QR code to view an example of a full COO job description and compensation package to use as a resource when you eventually hire for this position. Please note that compensation can vary based on experience, whether you engage a recruiter to hire externally for the role or if you are grooming and promoting someone from within your practice. For guidance on how to structure a fair compensation package, please reach out, and I will be happy to point you in the right direction.

Why the lengthy job description, you ask? Well, because it's a big job. This job description tells the candidate exactly what they should expect from working at this practice. It summarizes the person they're looking for to fulfill the role by using keywords about their core values.

Then, it outlines the salary and other benefits the role provides, which is something many companies refrain from doing. Here's a PSA to all companies: list your compensation range and benefits in your job description! This will not only showcase your company's transparency but also help you find candidates who are comfortable with those salary expectations.

The job description then lists the main tasks they will be responsible for, providing prospective candidates with a well-rounded picture of the role and how to succeed.

Finally, it outlines the background of the type of person they're looking for. Now, remember, this section is more like a wishlist. Obviously, very few people can have all the requirements listed in this section. But they should be meeting at least 70%. And while everything looks great on paper, it's important to remember that before you make any assumptions, you have to meet that person before you draw any conclusions. Since they'll be the person you're working closely with to put your vision forward, it's important that your core values and the DNA of your practice closely align with their thoughts, feelings, and motivations when joining your team.

Dr. Connor Despot recently hired his own COO to run his practice. He knew his main responsibility was patient care as an orthodontist, so by hiring a COO, he is now able to increase the number of patients he sees daily without getting burnt out by operational tasks:

> *"It's a huge investment to hire a COO. You take a big hit if you want to grow as a doctor because you have to pay them what they're worth, which comes right out of your pocket. But you hope that in a year or two down the road, that investment pays dividends. It's tough to do your job as an orthodontist while also managing all the ins and outs of everything. If you try to do it all, you run the risk of burning out, and then you're not going to reach your goals. So you have to be willing to make investments. I could physically see more than 100 patients daily, but now that I have a COO on board, it will allow me to see more if I need to."*

Now that you understand who your COO should be, why they're necessary for the growth of your practice, and what you can do to promote or hire one, let's now hear from a couple of COOs about the best practices they utilize to keep their offices' wheels churning like a well-oiled machine.

A Day In the Life of a COO

There are a lot of roles and responsibilities the COO must accomplish daily, as we know they are the ones who are accountable for bringing your vision to life. And as we've established, it's more like a partnership than an employer-employee relationship. However, your COO is still responsible for reporting any issues, changes, and resolutions back to you. You still have to have your eyes on your company and periodically check in to make sure your vision is being executed properly.

You have to put faith in your COO that they'll do a great job, but relinquishing all control is not in the cards. As the leader of the entire organization, you have to make sure your team is doing what they say they will be doing and hold them accountable for it. This doesn't mean you have to micro-manage, but you should be running quarterly meetings with your COO and leadership team to ensure they're doing everything you've laid out for them to full capacity.

But as for your leadership team, your COO is responsible for managing them. That is every director and manager you currently have running each department, like the director of sales, finance, marketing, patient care, operations, etc. It's like a domino effect. The way you inspire your COO is how they will inspire your leadership team. And the way your leadership team inspires your employees is how your employees will inspire patients. That's why clear messaging is so important. Because when the message isn't clear, your practice becomes a massive game of broken telephone, where every department relays a different message. Before you know it, your practice no longer has its core values intact.

It may seem like a huge responsibility because it is. You're not paying your COO six figures to sit around and look good. They have huge shoes to fill. So, what exactly does their day-to-day look like then? How can you ensure that you're setting your COO up for success as the manager of your leadership team? I reached out to Amanda Floyd from Fishbein Orthodontics and Janet Moser from AllSmiles Orthodontics to learn about their processes in managing multiple locations, departments, and teams as their practices' COO. Let's see what they had to say.

Amanda, what does a typical day look like for you as COO of Fishbein?

> *"I live by my calendar, and it's different every day. From the beginning, I've focused on building and maintaining our offices. We do everything from start to finish, from the designing to furnishing to building the schedule, putting the team in place, and hiring the right people. I'm also sitting in on meetings and interviews, discussing how our organization is structured. I work with each of the managers and then go down from there. Since our practice is so big, I have a person who works directly with me as our director of operations, so the whole leadership team reports to her, allowing me to focus on other major things in the business. We have different types of managers for each team. They all know whom they report to and who reports to them."*

Janet, how do you manage accountability?

> *"I learned quickly that you can't just trust people to say they're doing what they should be doing. You have to create a system of checks and balances to learn what is required of them, set the expectations for the job,*

and create checklists for reporting. Every position has a checklist they're responsible for sending to their direct report. You have to follow up on it with them continuously. Just because you've trained and coached them doesn't mean they will do it consistently if you're not following up. People respect what you inspect. And even if they're doing it right, everyone needs a refresher once in a while because people can get stuck in their habits. You're not there to micromanage, as no one likes that. However, if a job has to be done, there's a lot of responsibility and accountability that follows."

Amanda, how do you come up with your systems and processes? What do you use to document your systems?

"We have systems for everything. It looks straightforward now, but it didn't start that way. Two years ago, we didn't have a system for anything. So just little by little, as things have come up, you have to document what you're doing and what works for you, and then simplify it along the way. I constantly said, "It'd be easier if we had a checklist for this." So then we'd make one. We have a graphic designer that puts each checklist into a template so they all look the same. We must ensure every task is completed without needing to remember or recreate the wheel every time something happens."

Janet, how did the multiple departments and teams evolve?

"When creating multiple teams, there has to be someone in charge. So, the office manager is essentially the team leader. I train them, they train their team, and they report everything back to me. Since there are six locations that I'm responsible for, I have two teams in place that travel back and forth between locations. Each location is only *open part-time, so it works, and everyone helps each other out. Soon, thankfully, we'll be adding a third team and a third doctor. Since I have to manage all these locations, I'm trying to gear the culture toward three different teams. It's challenging, but everyone works hard, so I'm sure it'll be great."*

Amanda, Fishbein has probably gone through some of the most difficult growing pains I've encountered. Can you share some of the worst moments and how you overcame them?

"Rapid growth is hard to manage, especially if you don't expect it to reach that level. Staffing is the biggest issue because we don't want to hire just anyone. We do interviews almost every day, but out of the ten people we interview in a week, we'll just hire one. We're looking for the right personality fit. Then there's finding another doctor. We've grown so rapidly, and finding a doctor is even harder than finding a new front desk person. Then, you have to create more systems for all the growth you've had so you can maintain your culture. In the end, I think it's just finding the right mix of energy at each location and finding good team leaders to balance it out."

Everyone Has a Role to Play

Your COO will have a lot to manage daily, and every day will look different. Some days they might hire new staff and train, and other days they might deal with issues and put out fires. It's an ever-evolving job, and the person you put in this position needs to be aware of it and ready for the challenge. Luckily, Rome wasn't built in a day, and thousands of workers and leaders came together to create The Eternal City. Like your practice, your COO will have heaps of help from your leadership team. Now the question is, who's involved in this team? How big should this team be? How many departments do you need to have?

To answer these questions, you'll need to consider the level of growth you wish to attain because every level of growth looks different and involves various departments and teams to keep the business flowing smoothly and steadily. We'll thoroughly explain this in the next chapter, where I will discuss the small, medium, and large org charts your practice can use to plan your future team structure.

CHAPTER 3

Structuring Your Ideal Practice

When I released my first book, The Ultimate Practice, I felt a strong sense of accomplishment, knowing that I was finally getting the message out to hundreds of orthodontists who may have been struggling to understand their role as technicians while simultaneously being business owners. I had poured all of my insights into that book, and as brutally honest as I was, I thought the readers appreciated it. And for the most part, it was. But I'll never forget the day I received a phone call from one orthodontist.

She had read my book and immediately told me how offended she was. "What part offended you?" I asked her. "Well, in the title of Chapter 5, you tell orthodontists that they suck at doing business. That's not fair or true. I'm great at running my business," she responded accusingly.

The interesting thing about that was she had just started

her business. I tried to respond in the most polite way possible. "What can you show me to prove otherwise? Because from my understanding, the success of your business is yet to be determined, correct?" Shocked by my response, her rebuttal was, "Well, I can figure it out. It's not rocket science."

She had a point there—It's not rocket science. But here's the thing: running a business is a full-time job, and it takes a ton of work. I told her that if she looked past the chapter title, she would realize that the chapter talks about how an orthodontist is not trained to run a business; they're trained to fix patients' teeth and bite issues. But what you can do is hire someone whose experience is in running a business so that you can be an orthodontist full-time, doing five to ten thousand dollars an hour in production. Why split your time doing something you don't have any experience in and probably aren't that good at?

She was adamant that she could do it independently, so I left the conversation at that. Look, I'm not here to tell people they can't do it. I'm here to give people growth advice and explain what they can do to maximize their growth seamlessly without doing two full-time jobs (providing patient care and running a business) and without having zero time for a personal life outside of work.

And I get it. You're proud of what you've accomplished, and you want to make sure you have control over your business so you can protect its integrity. You want the best for yourself because you've worked hard to reach this point. Understandable. But I want you to know that it doesn't have to be so hard. It doesn't have to consume your whole life. Some people do their jobs exceptionally well, just as you are an orthodontics expert. Let those people in, and I promise you will feel a newfound sense of integrity and accomplishment within your business.

If you still feel like this orthodontist when reading this book, maybe this book is not for you. If you are interested in learning more about this, I'll share what some exceptional orthodontists I work with have accomplished by putting their egos aside and accepting help. Every great journey must begin with a vision and, of course, a map. Now, let's map out your ideal practice.

Org Charts: Why Are They So Important?

We know how important it is to document every single aspect of your vision for the proper execution to ensue. For that vision to come to life, you need a team, and every person's role must be mapped out on paper. You have to see where they fit in your practice, what their title will be, who they'll be reporting to, and who is accountable for them.

Think of your org chart as your accountability chart. Structuring this in a chart format is the most logical way to visually see how everything connects. As far as size goes, I have broken it down by production numbers which

I have arbitrarily defined as small, medium, and large practices [Disclaimer: this is my criteria, not necessarily the industry's]. Within each of these, you'll see the different roles and positions you'll need to develop and fill to move onto the next level.

• • •

Small Practice Org Chart

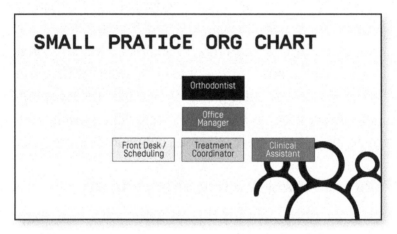

A small practice is defined as anything below three million in production. It consists of the orthodontist and the office manager as the leadership duo, responsible for the front desk and scheduling coordinator, treatment coordinator, and clinical assistant. You'll notice that this practice size doesn't require a COO, but it does have an office manager who would be running the day-to-day operations and reporting to the orthodontist. This is the stepping stone to getting to a medium-sized practice. So, if your practice isn't currently laid out this way, in that you don't have an office manager, this is where you first need to be in your growth journey.

Your office manager won't be the person making business decisions at this level—that'll still be you. But they will be able to do things like hire, fire, and manage your staff by providing the right direction. They're like your HR with busy work, leaving you with the time to run your business and take care of patients.

When looking for your office manager, you should look for similar qualities as described in the COO position regarding personality and attributes. This person needs to be able to lead a small team, think strategically, believe in your core values, and help execute them in your practice.

If you want to grow from a small to medium-sized practice, you should start thinking this way. You fill all the roles in the medium org chart with the people you have, so one person's responsibilities will fall into multiple roles. As you grow, you can shift them into more specialized roles and hire more people to fill the additional roles in the org chart. This is also how one person on your team can become well-versed in every role and take on more responsibility. If they have the ambition and drive and truly share your vision and core values, they may become ripe for grooming as the COO when you grow to the next level.

• • •

Medium Practice Org Chart

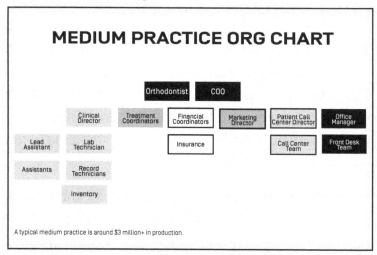

MEDIUM PRACTICE ORG CHART

| Orthodontist | COO |

- Clinical Director
- Treatment Coordinators
- Financial Coordinators
- Marketing Director
- Patient Call Center Director
- Office Manager

- Lead Assistant
- Lab Technician
- Insurance
- Call Center Team
- Front Desk Team

- Assistants
- Record Technicians

- Inventory

A typical medium practice is around $3 million+ in production.

A medium practice does between three and eight million in production. At this size, it's time to consider hiring a COO, as they'll be responsible for managing your leadership team. That's your clinical director, treatment coordinator, financial coordinator, marketing director, patient call center director, and office manager. Each of these individuals has their own departments to manage, and many of them will have their own team to manage, as well. While the orthodontist and COO are side-by-side in this chart at equal levels, it's important to note that the CEO and owner of the practice is the orthodontist. But when working in patient care at the office, they work under the COO, the operational leader.

Dr. Ernie McDowell, CEO of AllSmiles Orthodontics, said it best:

> "When I'm at the practice, I work under Janet [the COO]. When I'm not at the practice, or we're in a business meeting or conference, then she's reporting the day-to-day operations back to me. Other than that, she takes the lead."

Put That Ego Aside

If you want to grow to a medium-sized practice, you have to bring on a COO. When you bring on that COO, this is the mindset you need to have. Don't get me wrong, lots of doctors have grown to medium or large without one, but I do know that it is not the easiest, most efficient, and cost-effective way. It's time to put that ego aside and let your operational leader run your practice in your best interest.

That's probably Dr. Ben Fishbein's best trait: He doesn't have an ego. He lets the people he trusts take the lead without the need to micromanage, empowering team members to voice their opinions and call the shots. He doesn't yell or raise his voice when things go wrong. He takes the proper action to course correct as soon as issues transpire. That's probably why there's a unique synergy between him, his COO, and his leadership team. He knows when to step in and when to stay back. He's definitely a unicorn in this industry, as 95%

of orthodontists just can't allow themselves to do what he does with his team. It's unfortunate because when you step back and let your people shine, trust develops. That's how you're going to retain a strong team.

What If I Can't Afford It?

If you're still feeling concerned about the massive cost it'll be to bring on a COO, just think of it like this: Let's say you start them with a salary of 100K. Sure, that's a big hit because it comes right off your profits and take-home, but if you want to grow, it's your investment in your vision. Break it down. Each start is worth approximately $5000 to production. It would only take 20 new starts to pay for that salary. We have clients that have gotten more starts from a reactivation campaign. If you don't know how easy those are to do, revisit Book #2. Our best offices have no problem doing 20 starts in a week (or way beyond that). So there you have it. Salary paid. And as you continue to grow, offer your COO an annual performance bonus as the cherry on top to thank them for their successful contribution to that growth.

If you're running things at full capacity in a medium-sized practice, every single one of these people in this org chart is working to their full potential daily. The systems are in place, and everyone follows them, has someone to report to, and is held accountable for maintaining those standards. And if there are multiple locations, each one is consistent and efficient, with a brand and culture that looks the same.

It is only once you've perfected those systems and the teams within your org chart, in that they're working seamlessly through the motions and your schedule is at full capacity, that you can consider growing any further by opening another location. At this point, I'd like to point out that I've seen doctors grow to a large size with a single location.

Is It the Money or the Mission?

Some orthodontists are comfortable staying at the medium practice size. They enjoy bringing in five million in production annually and taking home two. They enjoy the lifestyle it brings them, going home in time for dinner with their family and playing golf on the weekends. But others seek out more from their positions as business owners. They want to provide their employees with opportunities to grow in this industry. They want to help people by providing free treatment and investing in their communities. That's why, when you're putting your vision onto paper, it's important to ask yourself this question: is it about the money, or is it about the mission?

If it's about the money, you're looking for a lifestyle practice. You want to be able to live the life you want, and the money from your practice will fund it. But if it's about the mission, then you're going to do everything in your power to grow as much as possible so you can reinvest that money into helping people.

That's a big job, and it's not for everyone. There's nothing wrong with wanting a lifestyle practice. Most of my clients have lifestyle practices, but some want to go above and beyond to fulfill a bigger mission. My goal with this book is to show more doctors that this is possible and increase the number of orthodontists inspired to grow to this level.

• • •

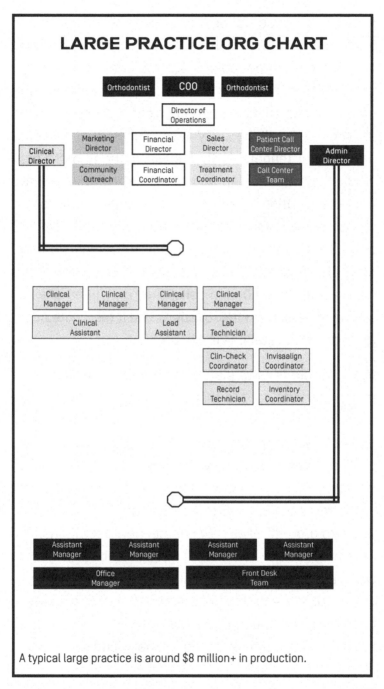

LARGE PRACTICE ORG CHART

| Orthodontist | COO | Orthodontist |

Director of Operations

Marketing Director	Financial Director	Sales Director	Patient Call Center Director
Clinical Director		Admin Director
Community Outreach	Financial Coordinator	Treatment Coordinator	Call Center Team

Clinical Manager	Clinical Manager	Clinical Manager	Clinical Manager
Clinical Assistant	Lead Assistant	Lab Technician
	Clin-Check Coordinator	Invisaalign Coordinator
	Record Technician	Inventory Coordinator

| Assistant Manager | Assistant Manager | Assistant Manager | Assistant Manager |
| Office Manager | Front Desk Team |

A typical large practice is around $8 million+ in production.

A large practice is anything over eight million in production. At this point, it's probably wise to bring another doctor on board, as you'll have too many patients to handle on your own, as well as a director of operations to help manage your leadership team, as your COO will be busy with higher-level business needs. Your leadership teams will manage more staff to keep up with the demand. Some large practices have multiple locations (Fishbein has 8, and AllSmiles has 6). Some key leadership roles in the org chart, like COO and Director of Marketing, are centralized, while other roles are duplicated in each location. If the practice has centralized their inbound calls, they only need one call center to service all the locations. We'll talk more about locations and satellites in Chapter 7.

Many people tend to plateau at the eight-million dollar mark when they get to this practice size. They've done everything right up until now, adding all the necessary roles and departments to reach their goals. But like every other journey aspect, it begins with your mindset. What gets you to one level will not work to get you to the next level. You can't just do more of what you were always doing to grow. It takes new people, new operations, and new procedures. You should be clear about what you want and the people you will involve to help get you there. You have to think BIG. And one person's ability to think big is not enough. You need a team of people, both internally and externally, who will help lead you there.

That's why, to achieve a large practice producing well beyond eight million, you need to up your internal marketing and hire an external marketing team (such as HIP!) to get your name out there. You need a community outreach coordinator to go out and deliver your message to new people. You need to sponsor and make your brand known to the masses. You need people to immediately think of you when they think of orthodontic treatment. You'll need to duplicate your team in one location and another. You need all the help you can get, and you need to be comfortable investing the money, as it's the best investment you'll make as a business owner on a mission for greatness.

Dr. Ed Wentz owns an eight-figure practice in Texas, and at 65 years old, he's still hungry for more.

I'll never forget a story his COO, Joe, told me during a dinner we had a few years back. He shared how during one month, his team was able to achieve 400 starts. When Ed heard this, he immediately said, "Wow, 400 starts. That's great. Why don't we do 500 next?"

When I heard that, I couldn't help but think about what Magic Johson said after he purchased an investment company and brought it from 14 billion to 20 billion dollars:

> *"Let's celebrate for five minutes and then get back to work."*

I laughed and told him that's a visionary mindset. Joe

continued, explaining how it's hard for him to fathom more growth because they're constantly putting in 100% of their effort, and he always wants more. He explained how they would have to hire five more people to reach 500 starts. Ed's response? "So? Hire five more people, then!"

That's the ultimate difference between the visionary and the integrator: The integrator often can't think that big and sometimes finds it hard to understand. In the integrator's mind, they're thinking of every nuanced detail and the possible changes they'll need to make to achieve that. The visionary isn't thinking of the steps they need to implement to make it happen or how much it will cost them. But that's what you want. You want that visionary to always want more. More for themselves and more for others. It's meeting a goal and setting a higher goal right after. It's always striving for the next phase. For visionaries like Ed, the mission never ends. The mindset is always to improve. And as difficult as it may be for the COO to understand, they will put forth that vision to the best of their ability when they have a leader that truly believes it is possible. That balance is necessary when running a successful business, resulting in a healthy relationship between the COO and CEO.

Managing Accountability

In the previous chapter, Janet, the COO at AllSmiles, mentioned that holding your team accountable to the responsibilities outlined in their designated roles is not just something that can be taught once and left up to their own devices. Their respective managers and directors should always be checking in, following up, training, and coaching in the necessary areas. Amanda, the COO at Fishbein, reinforces this by saying the team is responsible for following each procedure. Managing accountability is extremely important if you want longevity in the success of your business. Knowing what the chain of command is, from your bottom line to your top line, should be clear and consistent. You should be hiring, firing, recognizing, and rewarding your team based on these behaviors. By not doing this, certain aspects of your practice will crumble and fall apart. You will risk having unhappy patients and employees and a negative reputation within your community.

Managing accountability starts with you, and it is passed onto your leadership team to maintain daily. It starts with you outlining the behaviors and expectations you expect from your COO, your COO demonstrating them to the leadership team, and the leadership team relaying them to the rest of your staff. It's an ongoing process, but by staying consistent, your entire staff will be working towards meeting your goals in the most efficient way possible.

Dr. Fishbein recalls when he only had 20 employees working at his practice. He now has a team of over 100 employees, so he knows there are a lot of people responsible for various tasks and many leaders responsible for making sure those tasks are completed at the highest standard. But he also knows that when one person slacks and doesn't do their part, everyone else can feel it:

> "You can have the best treatment coordinator (TC) in the world, but if your scheduling coordinator doesn't answer the phone, the TC won't be able to make that sale. Every role is incredibly important, from the doctor to the person answering the phone, because if there's one misstep, it'll almost throw the whole thing off. As you grow, I think it's important that you have those team members in place who are ready to take on those responsibilities, and their managers are ready to hold them accountable because otherwise, you'll just hinder your growth."

Can You Make It Your Reality?

Growing from small to medium to large can be lengthy and time-consuming, but with the right commitment, dedication, and buy-in from your team, the journey of getting there can be quite rewarding. However, the only way you will build a team who can meet the expectations you've set out for them is by first creating a successful brand and a welcoming culture that is conducive for them to thrive and grow. In the next chapter, we'll outline how you can promote your brand, showcase your culture, and uphold and maintain them to allow your vision and core values to shine fully within your practice and community.

CHAPTER

4

Manifesting Your Brand and Culture Through Marketing

In this day in age, we are surrounded by companies that provide similar product offerings and services. If I want a coffee, there are dozens of coffee shops in my neighborhood I could walk into to get one. If I want a pair of shoes, there are hundreds of retailers I could visit either in-store or online to buy a new pair. But let's be honest. You don't want to pick between dozens of coffee shops and hundreds of retailers. Because it's hard having so many options—how do you know which one you'll like? Ultimately, you will gravitate toward the company whose brand and culture are the strongest. So when you want a coffee, you might automatically think of a Starbucks latte, or when you want a new pair of shoes, a fresh pair of Nikes may fulfill that desire. Your brand has to be so strong that when people think of getting orthodontic treatment, they think of you first.

What's the Difference Between Your Brand and Culture?

Your brand and culture are the pinnacles of your success as a profitable business. Some businesses put so much emphasis on the products and services they provide but then neglect to sell people on who they are as a company: what their values are, what they believe in, the type of people they want working for them, the types of behaviors and personalities they want interacting with the world.

Your brand is a perception, and that perception is associated with visual images that help bring it to life. It's the logo affiliated with your name. It's the products and services that come to mind when they see your logo. It's how people feel when they think about your products and services. It's all of these little details that people see that allow them to automatically know it's you and, in turn, feel positively about that.

Your culture, on the other hand, is your core values brought to life by your employees and delivered to your patients to create a positive experience. You can't have a successful brand if you don't have a successful culture. The two go hand-in-hand. You need a strong office culture with happy employees, which creates happy patients and leaves you with a positive brand name. To achieve that, you need to be a CEO with a clear vision and strong core values, have a COO who believes in those values, and develop a leadership team to enable your employees to bring them to the forefront. Each of these individuals must consistently ensure that your brand is reflected in your culture so the rest of the world knows what you stand for.

What Does It Look Like?

A small practice averaging 1.2 in production has the standard run-of-the-mill approach to marketing. They probably have a couple of dentists referring patients to their office, or they're sponsoring one or two schools. They most likely run print or digital ads now and then and have a mediocre website that outlines brief information about their practices' location and services. The problem with this marketing approach is it's not strategic enough to make it work like a well-oiled machine. These practices are not using the potential that marketing can do for them, and it's ultimately preventing their growth.

You don't want to be one of these practices, so you decide to invest in the proper marketing services to create brand awareness in your community. Let's say you did a bunch of things to get it started. You put out your digital marketing ads, rented billboards in your community, improved your website, and even hired a marketing director and a marketing/community outreach coordinator to perform your internal marketing and community outreach. Your coordinator starts interacting with dental practices in the community by donating gift baskets with your logo and informing them that your practice is accepting new patients at your office down the road. The dentists instantly buy into her elevator pitch and start referring your practice to their patients who are candidates for orthodontic treatment.

Amazing! You just got a bunch of warm prospective patients referred because of an amazing effort to get your brand out there. But then, your COO notices that a few prospective patients referred from the dental clinic came in for consultations and never ended up starting treatment. He asks your treatment coordinator why they never started, to which she shakes her head and replies, "I'm not sure."

He decides to dig a little deeper and look at your Google reviews. You notice some of the latest reviews are pretty negative:

> "Too pushy. I came in for a consultation, and they kept convincing me to start that same day when I wasn't ready to. Won't be coming back."

> "Didn't feel very welcomed when I came in. Staff didn't seem prepared and could barely answer my questions."

> "When I was in the waiting room, I heard the front desk people talking badly about some of their patients. I could overhear their entire conversation. Not impressed and will not be returning."

Extremely infuriated, he informs your office manager, who manages the front desk and scheduling team, about these reviews. She's not sure what to say, only that she will try to talk to the team to understand what happened.

Three prospective patients that could have started chose not to because of the horrible service they received from your team. They're probably not very thrilled with the dentist who referred them, and they're going to tell everyone they know about the horrible experience they had.

What's the message here? While marketing and community outreach are essential, they're not serving you if you can't even nail down the fundamentals of exuding a positive culture in your workplace. No amount of gift baskets, donuts, or sponsorships will save you. Your brand can only shine if it has the culture to back it up—that begins with excellent customer service. Once your team consistently thrives in that area and makes the patient experience a memorable one, then you can feel confident putting your name and logo out there and jump-starting your community outreach.

To learn how to get started and eventually master your community outreach, scan here to watch this interview with Lori Harris, Community Outreach Coordinator at Fishbein Orthodontics.

The Face of Your Practice: Marketing Your Brand and Logo

Your logo is the simple visual people will remember you by. Think of all the brands you currently love. Does their logo automatically come to mind when you think of them? You could probably recall 80% of them right now. When designing your logo, you should ensure it's smart, memorable, and representative of your practice.

Take Fishbein Orthodontics, for example. Dr. Fishbein used his name to his advantage and made his logo a fish named Chompers. Chompers even has braces! He even went further and personified Chompers, making him the mascot during their events. When Dr. Fishbein promotes his practice, what people constantly see is Chompers, the fish. The Fishbein Orthodontics brand is now everywhere in their community: on T-shirts, in the humane society, during bridal events, and on boxes of donuts. He's the smile provider for their local baseball stadium, The Pensacola Wahoos, and the minor league hockey team, The Pensacola Ice Flyers. He's infiltrated all the schools, created a non-profit organization to give away free smiles to bullied kids, has billboards all over town, and has been the topic of local news on multiple occasions. Everywhere you go in town, you see the fish of Fishbein Orthodontics. When people think about getting orthodontic treatment in that area, they immediately think and go to Fishbein. That's the power your brand and logo can have.

Only some people can do this. Dr. Fishbein went into significant debt to put his name and logo out there to the extent he did. He took his branding to the next level because he knew he would reap the benefits of it afterward. Dr. Fishbein has been in business for almost ten years, and his journey is a notable one. It wasn't easy, but he had a vision and a plan to execute it. He was in it for the mission. He could only achieve his massive level of success because he had a strong foundation, a positive work culture, and a team who continuously bought into his vision.

Fishbein's Director of Marketing, Aliza Ray, spoke to me about the importance of marketing the brand through multiple channels and explained why it's necessary to take on smart debt if you're trying to grow your practice:

> "The biggest mistake some orthodontists make is not spending money on marketing. If you want to make money, you have to spend money. That's the only way you're going to grow. The thing that we did was not say 'no.' If we were approached to do an event or campaign, we automatically said we would try it. Why not? If it comes back negative, we won't do it next time. If it comes back positive, we'll put more money into it to make it better going forward. It took a bit of back and forth; we made some mistakes. We did an expensive commercial for the local movie theater, which didn't work out so well, haha... We learned our lesson a few times the hard way, but it will always make up for itself in the end, if not tenfold."

To listen to the full interview with Aliza, scan this QR code.

SCAN ME

Only some have the means to do this when they first start off or even years down the road. You have to first focus on the fundamentals of strengthening your brand and culture internally through your patient experience and then slowly work toward showcasing them to the rest of the world.

Dr. Kristen Knecht from Knecht Orthodontics is a prime example of this. We started working with her about two years ago when she had just graduated and opened up her practice. From the get-go, she did everything the right way. She created a great brand, perfected her website, nailed the customer experience, and scaled her marketing. She and her team started going to events in the community and increased their digital marketing by working with HIP. Dr. Knecht used a similar approach as Dr. Fishbein but on a smaller scale. She's not going into as much debt to do it and is experiencing growth a little slower, but she's still growing ten times faster than most orthodontic practices.

It All Begins With a Budget

You have to know how much smart debt you can take on if you plan to hire people to fulfill your internal and external marketing and community outreach within your practice. You can't just spend, spend, and spend beyond your means. So, I've outlined a list of steps for your marketing team (alongside the COO) to implement so they understand where to start and how to stay on track:

Step 1: Create a budget to work within.

Step 2: Make a spreadsheet, start to map out everything, and add it up.

Step 3: Make a calendar with all of the activities.

Step 4: Execute.

Step 5: Measure.

This is Fishbein Orthodontics' internal marketing and outreach calendar. There's nothing like a gigantic, color-coded calendar in your staff room to keep your team organized and on track!

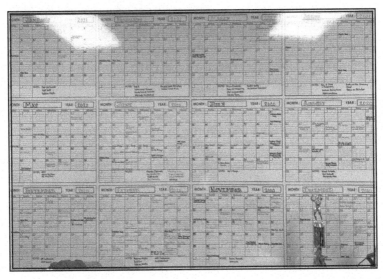

Let's Hear From the Experts!

I interviewed CEOs and COOs we currently partner with to conduct research for this book, wanting to understand their steps to improve their brand and culture. Here's what they had to say:

Dr. Despot, how did you develop your brand, and how is that reflected in your locations?

> "We just looked at who we were as a team. We knew we were fun, family-oriented, and flexible. We knew we only wanted positive vibes. One of our sayings is, "Straight teeth and positive vibes"—that's what our brand is. You can't come up with a brand that's not you, or people will see straight through that. You can only fake it for so long before the truth comes out. It's best just to be yourself and run with that. In our locations, the music's pumping every day, and it's bright and inviting. We're always joking around and laughing, and we spend a little extra time chatting with the patients. It's too frequent that you go somewhere and no one talks to you or even calls you by your first name—there's no interaction or human touch. We didn't want that, so we're heavy on the interactions. We ask folks how their days are going and what's new in their lives. That's how I want people to remember us."

Dr. Fishbein, what's the secret to having a good workplace culture?

> "There's no secret to it. When your team members are happy, you can feel it. They're happy for a reason—you can't fake happiness when working with people for eight hours a day. You have to give your staff a reason to show up to work every day. Whether through incentives

like bonuses or promotions to reward their hard work or just having a great group of people they enjoy being around daily. You can't magically have a positive work culture if you don't have positive employees. You can feel that energy when you walk into any business. When the culture isn't good, you can see the employees don't want to be there."

Janet, how have you developed a healthy culture within your team?

"When we're hiring, we love warm referrals. If you know someone that wants to work with us, we welcome them to come to join us and be a part of our team. We like using that approach because our team knows our core values and the types of personalities we welcome at our office. If they have friends who believe in and embody those values, we feel more comfortable corresponding with them first before we look externally. We also try to incentivize the team, so there are team bonuses and outings that we do after work or on the weekends to let loose. For example, we have an upcoming staff appreciation night at the race stadium, and we rented the bullpen box. We have our vision and core values that we try to adhere to every day, so we continuously strive to maintain that culture. Seeing that helps them understand who Dr. McDowell (AllSmiles' CEO) is and how he wants to be represented in the community."

Amanda, what makes your office culture different?

"Part of it is because we have an awesome CEO (Dr. Fishbein) who's super laid back, loves music, and is open to all our ideas for the office. The other part is we are focused on the patient experience. Our staff is always *smiling, and if one of them is having a bad day, I just let them go home. We're always overstaffed, so I don't want anyone to work if they're not feeling it that day. Our office has a relaxed-at-home vibe, like you're visiting somebody's house for coffee—it's far from commercial-looking and differs from traditional orthodontic practices. We have a wall that has every single patient's photo on it. We have photoshoots about once a quarter for patients that are coming out of treatment, and we've recently started implementing people that are still in treatment, which is kind of fun for them. We have Dippin' Dots, drinks, and other snacks at every location for whoever wants them. The music is fast and upbeat to get everyone pumped for the day. The patients love it, the parents love it, and the team loves it. What more could you want? We just want to make everyone happy and enjoy being here."*

It's All About Your People

It's easy to notice that the common theme in each of the responses you've just read is to have the right people in place to promote the culture you envision for your practice. Without the right people in the right seats, you'll never achieve a positive culture and a strong brand. You must put 100% of your efforts into finding the right people who believe in your vision and core values and maintaining standards by consistently training, coaching, and rewarding those valuable team players. In the next chapter, we'll discuss how you can find the right talent, fill the right seats, and create a positive candidate and employee experience to amplify your practice's brand and culture.

CHAPTER

5

Attracting the Right People for the Right Seats

A while back, one of my clients told me about the COO they hired to run their practice. After a few months of working with this person, they realized he had fabricated the entire interview process and hid behind the mask of an elite expert in operations. Once he had to deliver on his talk, the mask fell away, revealing that he was not what he had portrayed himself. On top of it all, he started to rub the entire team the wrong way. He was rude, egotistical, sexist, and basically a creep.

This team had worked very hard to implement systems and procedures with accountability and ownership for results. They thought they were taking the next logical step in their growth by adding the role of the COO. They had been growing consistently and continued to see an increase in production after he came on board. Even though he had only been with the team for three months, he tried to take the credit for a 35% increase in production while leaving a path of destruction in his wake.

He claimed to be able to negotiate insurance contracts that would provide generous reimbursements. Upon further scrutiny, what he was suggesting was insurance fraud. He boasted connections with oral surgery centers which later denied having any affiliation with him. He talked poorly about staff members behind their backs and on one occasion, blatantly called the doctor's sister-in-law stupid. One team member quit, citing him as her reason for leaving. In her exit interview, she mentioned that six other team members were thinking of quitting because of him, as well. He actually went as far as touching a woman's backside during a community event. Luckily, there were witnesses.

Not only had he wreaked havoc on the practice from the inside, but he had also managed to tarnish the brand to the public. After dealing with all these unfortunate events, he was terminated shortly thereafter.

The Onboard Terrorist

This insufferable COO is an over-the-top example of what we call an "onboard terrorist." This is someone who hijacks your office with negative attitudes and toxic behaviors, ultimately ruining the culture you and your team work so hard to build.

The first time I heard this term was during an interview

I did with David Staughton, a business consultant who works with plastic surgeons in Australia. This is how he describes the onboard terrorist:

> "Someone in your practice who is absolutely killing your practice. It can be the wicked person at the front desk. It could be the practice manager. It could be the nurse. There's somebody in there that just doesn't want to do it and is literally limiting and minimizing your practice. They are your onboard terrorist who is stopping your practice from growing."

Most of the time, this person will make little to no effort to change and continue to tarnish relationships and ignore procedures, despite multiple retraining attempts. Often, they are someone that you feel is indispensable. They want you to feel this way and that's exactly how they hold you hostage. You may have inherited them when you took over a practice. They could be running the whole show and you worry that if they left, all the knowledge would go out the door with them. No matter what you try to do to convince yourself that they are helping your practice, something always feels off. The worst thing you can do for your business is to keep an onboard terrorist on board.

You have to keep a lookout for these people because they are like a cancer in your office. They take more than their fair share of energy and give nothing in return. Some are terminal if they are not removed immediately, but many go unnoticed for long periods before the damage they are causing is discovered.

Another practice we worked with appeared to be crushing it for a while. Their marketing was working brilliantly until it wasn't. One day the doctor called me and said, ``Hey Luke, my production is tanking.'' It didn't make sense. When we started looking into things a little deeper we found out that they were not following up with leads and no one on the team was taking any accountability for the processes we had shown them for responding to and converting the leads we generated.

It turned out that the office manager wasn't holding team members accountable. She was more interested in the team liking her than leading them. We had to dig in, create some systems, create an org chart for them and encourage her to train teams to be specialists vs generalists. As soon as we started holding her accountable she quit. Three other team members followed her out the door.

We helped the doctor hire and train the right team members and now he is thriving. While it can be painful to fire someone, it has to be done. You simply can't allow people to hijack your vision and destroy your practice.

If you've found yourself in a similar situation, you're not alone. Most practices will struggle with an onboard terrorist at one point or another. This person could be absolutely anyone from the treatment coordinator to the director of operations. Regardless of who it is, take action quickly. Holding on always leads to a toxic workplace environment and tanked conversion rates.

I'm currently dealing with an eight-figure practice, but this year, they're down by three million in production. They've blamed it on staffing since they missed 50% of calls. The COO complained that they couldn't find quality people to do the scheduling coordinating role because they refuse to work for $14 per hour—all of them want a minimum of $18 per hour. My response? Well, just pay them $18 per hour. You're an eight-figure practice closing on dozens of starts per day at $5,000 each, and you can't pay your scheduling staff a liveable wage? It's not rocket science. Times have changed, inflation is through the roof, and it's tough to live in this economy. People aren't going to feel motivated to do their job if they're barely scraping by.

Unfortunately, this COO has limiting beliefs that are not serving his staff or the practice's growth. He doesn't believe this solution is what will allow them to maintain their eight-figure practice. So they won't, and they'll continue to lose quality people because they can't wrap their heads around the reality we're currently living in. If I were the CEO, I would probably coach this individual and break down the obstacles so we could move forward together. If that doesn't work, I would start looking for a new COO.

So, it comes down to these questions: How can you ensure you're going through the proper hiring and onboarding process to avoid bringing on an onboard terrorist? Are your roles adequately defined and laid out in an accountability chart? Do you have procedures for training and evaluation that ensure that an employee is measuring up to their role and delivering? In this chapter, we'll address these questions and demonstrate the right processes to adhere to when hiring, training, evaluating and terminating. This will help you attract the right candidates who fully align with your core values and contribute to the positive culture in your practice.

Creating a Thriving Ecosystem

Like an evolving ecosystem, everything within your practice must integrate harmoniously—from your core values to your processes and your people—to prosper. You need people who will create a positive culture, but you also need a workplace environment where your people can thrive. Many moving parts occur simultaneously to make this happen. Still, it's not difficult to achieve if you and your team are actively sticking to your vision and implementing your core values. As Dr. Fishbein said in the previous chapter, you have to give your staff a reason to come to work every day, but you also need staff who deliver to their full capacity every time. It's this interchangeable relationship where you can't have one without the other. So, if you want a thriving ecosystem, it's best to either get rid of the organism that has the capability of dissolving it completely or, better yet, prevent it from entering in the first place! This is why your hiring process is essential for the success of your practice. Get it right the first time around, and eliminate threats that tarnish your ecosystem.

Breaking Down the Hiring Process

Who's Doing the Hiring?

If you have a small practice, you are probably responsible for hiring your employees, but if you intend to grow as a medium or even large-sized practice, you should get your COO to take over the hiring process. If you have other departments and roles in place and a COO knowledgeable in each of those departments and roles, it should be an area they can excel in because they know the exact responsibilities a prospective candidate must be able to fulfill. So, ensure your COO reads this section of the book as well, as it's written specifically for you and them!

Where Should You Source Your Candidates From?

Many of the nation's leading orthodontic practices, like Fishbein and AllSmiles, mostly rely on warm referrals when looking to hire for their departments. This is a great approach because you would be getting those referrals from your already beloved staff or family members, who may have someone in mind whom they believe aligns with your practice's core values like they do.

Amanda from Fishbein has compiled a team where over 90% of the staff were hired based on warm referrals:

> "We hire strictly based on warm referrals. The 90% that I've hired have been from them knowing someone who works here, or they had a friend or family member who is or was a patient who referred them to us. The other 10% have been from people I've come across from other establishments. Literally, if I receive great customer service from someone, I'll give them my business card and tell them if they want to change their profession to give me a call."

Warm referrals are a great method, but they aren't always as successful as Amanda's experience. Therefore, you should have other options available when looking to hire, such as posting a job description on a job board site like Indeed, LinkedIn, or ZipRecruiter. You will be fishing in a bigger pond, so it's important to make sure your job descriptions are as detailed as possible, outlining the key responsibilities, attributes, and experience you're looking for to find a handful of ideal candidates to interview.

Review the COO job description in Chapter 2 if you'd like to see an example of what this description should look like. But like most things in life, it's great to have someone to guide you through it. If you want to source the right candidates for your practice, consider reaching out to Wiseman Strategies. They provide a guided service to help employers find the right talent to reduce turnover, increase retention, and improve engagement. HIP partnered with them a couple of years ago, and they've helped us—and many of our orthodontic partners—hire several of our talented staff members since then.

I spoke to Tony Wiseman, CEO of Wiseman Strategies, about sourcing the right candidates when hiring talent for your business. Here's what he had to say:

> "When you do the appropriate work ahead of time and assess the job itself, you get targeted language you can put in a job posting that calls out to the right candidate to apply. You need to write a captivating hook, determine what the job stimuli are and how someone will respond to that, and think about the words themselves—what you say and how you say it says a lot about what you want and care about. So, you need to be proactive in the way that you post but also in what you post. It's also a great idea to ask candidates in the description to send an introductory video of themselves. It'll help you get to know the person beyond their resume."

I have to say, the introductory video works. We've been asking for introductory videos from our prospective candidates at HIP since I initially heard this from Tony, mostly because the ones that are not serious about the position just won't include a video, which means you can easily toss their resumes aside. Focus on the candidates who did send in a video—they're the ones that are interested in the role.

Even billionaire Richard Branson believes in this method! In his MasterClass, he asserts that just by receiving a 5-minute video from a candidate, "you'll be able to see a lot of their personality—you're going to see whether they're smiling or if they've got some oomph!"

 To learn more about Wiseman Strategies Guided Services, scan this QR code.

So you've compiled your list of prospective candidates using this approach, and they all look good. Now...

How Should You Prepare for the Interview?

Remember the Predictive Index (PI)? Of course, since I've shown you numerous examples in Front Desk Secrets, The Ultimate Treatment Coordinator, and earlier on in this book. At this point, it's best to get your candidates to complete a PI assessment of their own. It'll help you assess behavioral aspects of the role and determine how your candidate is most likely to perform, if they are in alignment, if there's a gap, or if they have the right coping mechanisms to address their weaknesses. Ultimately, it will help you understand if the person will be able to assimilate with the culture of your practice.

In the meantime, you should be coming up with a list of questions that address the person as a whole. You want to find out who they are, what they like, what their short- and long-term goals are, and why they want to work for you. You want to ensure they're the right fit for your practice. But this is what many practices forget to ask: is your practice the right fit for them?

So, consider this: Before you start the Q&A part of the interview, it may be wise to have the candidate watch a presentation about your practice. Include who you are, your history, your backstory, your core values and DNA, your customers (or patients), and your expertise. You can make a slide deck to include a presentation summary, including keywords, phrases, and photos. It doesn't have to be very long: 15 to 30 minutes would do the trick. It's about selling them on your mission and what you stand for. Your candidates will appreciate the transparency you've given them, and if they're the right fit, they'll buy into it, and it will be easier to move on with the interview process. So, spend the time to create this before the interview.

Scan here to see the slide deck HIP uses in our hiring process!

How Do You Create a Great Interview Experience?

Before we go over each interview phase in detail, I've outlined some key things to consider to create a great interview experience. Be sure to apply these during the two interview phases:

- Be prepared in advance and remain consistent (i.e., have your slide deck and questions ready for each candidate).

- Before the interview, explain to each candidate how the interview will go as it will help set clear expectations, maintain structure, and diffuse nervous energy.

- Make sure you stick to your questions and avoid bringing things up that can be a concern for discrimination (i.e., don't ask about their age, sexual preferences, political stance, or religion).

- When interviewing candidates, use a scoring card or matrix to compare them equally without bias.

- Discern if the candidate is the right fit for your practice (i.e., the role, team, culture, etc.).

- Determine if their strengths will allow them to do the job well and if you can train their gaps.

Let's say you want to conduct two interviews with your prospective candidates. You've compiled a handful of resumes that align best with the job description, and a few of them have even sent introductory videos of themselves and have described what excites them about the role and your practice. Those people have a great demeanor, an impressive resume, and confidence that you see working for your practice. You decide you want to start the interview process with them, so you send them the PI assessment to complete before their first interview.

The First Interview

Your first interview is about getting to know the candidate and them getting to know you. You can easily do this by setting up a video call via Zoom, where you can showcase your brief presentation about your company and ask your preliminary questions to the candidate. This will allow the candidate to find out about your company and decide if you're the right workplace for them. Similarly, it will give you an idea if they'd be the right fit for your culture and brand identity.

For your questions, you'll want to keep it light since you're getting to know the person. Start with some introductory questions, ask about their experience, dive into the role they've applied for, and ask more specific questions, like:

- Can you tell me a bit about yourself?
- Why do you want to work for our company?
- What are your salary expectations?
- Why are you leaving your current role?
- How do you run meetings?
- How would you set expectations for team members and manage resources?
- Can you tell me about a situation when you had to implement something new?
- Is there a situation when you had to accomplish multiple objectives under a tight timeline?
- If we were to make an offer, what's your timeline?

If you're satisfied with their answers, proceed to the second interview.

The Second Interview

The second interview is where you'll ask some of the harder questions, like:

- What is your greatest strength?
- What is the toughest decision you ever had to make?
- How comfortable are you with terminating someone if needed?
- How do you perform under pressure?
- How do you hope or plan to shield the owners of the company long-term?
- How hard will you work in your first 90 days to get up to speed to assist in running the company?
- How do you plan to understand what we do and how we work to effectively manage the team?

When you've reached the end of the process, consolidate the notes you've taken into a document. Include the person's general information, the results of their PI assessment, and notes about the questions asked and answers received from the first and second interviews. Evaluate the documents fairly and decide who gets the role. By this point, you should feel confident with your decision and excited to begin the onboarding process!

Scan these QR codes to see an example of this document and to listen to a second interview with me and a prospective candidate who applied for a marketing position with HIP [FYI, she got the job!].

Unveiling the Onboarding Process

Congrats! You've gone through the entire interview process from beginning to end. If you've done it correctly, you're probably feeling super confident about your new hire. You've provided a successful candidate experience that will hopefully turn into a successful employee experience. But to make sure your new hire is on the road towards a successful employee experience, you need to equip and prepare them from the start, and that begins with your onboarding process. Your onboarding process needs to be just as smooth as your hiring process for that new hire to shine.

Breaking Down the Onboarding Process

Who's Doing the Training?

At this point, your new hire should already have a clear understanding of your history, core values, DNA, and mission, and a brief idea about what to expect from their role and the responsibilities required to perform the role successfully. But other than that, they're a blank canvas waiting to be turned into a masterpiece. The way they are trained from this point forward is a direct reflection of their future success. So, if they're trained poorly, they'll perform poorly. It's probably best to get one of your more seasoned staff members to do the training from here on out. As you or your COO have been heavily involved in the hiring process, it's time to relinquish the reins and get back to the other pressing tasks you need to do to run your business!

Janet from AllSmiles is involved in the hiring process from the initial job post to the moment the candidate is hired, but that journey ends on their first day:

> "I'll do everything with them up until their first day. Then, the team lead (office manager) takes over. They can either train the new hire themselves if they have the time or get a seasoned staff member who's knowledgeable of each role and department to do it. They'll get them to fill out the onboarding forms, set them up with the online training, go over each of the checklists, shadow different roles within the practice, and schedule them for weekly check-ins to provide feedback. All our new hires have a

four-week training checklist they have to complete and submit to me for review, so that's only when I enter into the picture again."

Which Resources Should You Use to Train?

If you're an established practice, you most likely already have many up-to-date training manuals and checklists to help get your new hires started. But it can sometimes feel a bit daunting to dive head first into a manual that outlines everything they're responsible for. So, instead, ease them into the process with a series of videos to help get them started.

One thing I recommend to all our clients is to have their new staff take HIP's Ultimate Training Guide. There are dozens of videos applicable to a variety of departments and roles. We have ones dedicated to your front desk and scheduling coordinators, your treatment coordinators, your marketing team, and even ones for your director of operations and COOs. The videos provide a general overview of navigating the position effectively, allowing your new hires to get a sound idea of how to perform early in the onboarding process.

In addition to that, we also have a whole section dedicated to PracticeBeacon (PB), organized in a way that will walk your new hire through the entire system. Depending on their role, you can also get them to read Front Desk Secrets and The Ultimate Treatment Coordinator (and this book, too, if you've hired a Director of Operations or COO to run your practice), as it will provide them with practical tools such as systems, processes, and best practices to get them right on track. And before you know it, they will have settled into the role quite seamlessly.

You'll have access to the complete set of videos in the Ultimate Training Guide by scanning this QR code.

All you have to do is submit your email address, name, and phone number, and you'll receive unlimited access to our training modules so you can provide the ultimate training experience to your new employees.

How Do You Track Their Progress?

Tracking the progress of every new hire is essential if you want to ensure they're assimilating into the role well. Letting small mistakes go unnoticed for too long can turn into mayhem, so ensure your team catches them early and continuously coaches to improve and accelerate their progress. There are a few things your team will want to pay attention to, such as:

- Are they catching on quickly?

- Are they asking the right questions?
- Are they learning from their mistakes?
- Are they eager to learn more?
- Are they visibly excited to show up to work?
- Are they going above and beyond?

If you can confidently say 'yes' to all of these questions, your team is on the right track to move forward. But if they're not, it's important to let your team know to raise these concerns early so you can nip them in the bud at the onset. Habits are harder to break down the road, and you definitely don't want an onboard terrorist situation!

True Leadership Is Key

Ultimately, your new hire will only thrive in their new role if they have the proper leadership to help them succeed. You empower your leaders, and they empower your staff. I often recall an excerpt from Napoleon Hill's classic book, Think and Grow Rich, when I think about what it means to be a true leader. In the book, he concludes that successful leaders tend to think and act similarly. To back up his statement, he outlines 11 major attributes he believes all leaders have in common after observing 25,000 successful people over a 25-year timeframe. These include:

1. Unwavering Courage
2. Self-Control

3. A Keen Sense of Justice

4. The Definitiveness of Decision

5. The Definitiveness of Plans

6. The Habit of Doing More Than Paid For

7. A Pleasing Personality

8. Sympathy and Understanding

9. Mastery of Detail

10. Willingness to Assume Full Responsibility

11. Cooperation

When your leadership team exemplifies each of these major attributes, it won't go unnoticed by your staff. Quite the contrary. Your staff will begin to embody these attributes and grow into a leader themselves. When that kind of confidence and assurance consistently surrounds you, it's contagious. My team at HIP decided to create our version of these attributes. They are written on our break room whiteboard to remind us of our commitment to whom we need to be every time we come to work.

• • •

1. Stay in the details
2. Be willing to do everything that I delegate
3. Expect to be paid for what I DO (not know)
4. Not afraid of subs rising to my level
5. Great imagination
6. Selfless (needs no honor)
7. temperate
8. loyal
9. leads by encouragement, sympthy. understanding
10. Needs no title

It's Time to Measure Your Growth!

Now that you have sourced the right people for the right seats, you can successfully showcase your brand and culture to the rest of the world. It's an exciting time, usually when proper growth starts. Your name is out there, and people are hearing the buzz. Your phones are getting busier, and your staff is working to their total capacity. The more you grow, the more intense this will become. Are you ready for it? I'm sure you are because that's why you're reading this! But do you know how to correctly track, measure, and report all of this newfound growth? Do you know what it takes to do this daily, weekly, and monthly? Don't worry if this is new to you because that's what we'll discuss in the next chapter.

CHAPTER 6

Reporting and Measuring Your Growth

"What gets measured gets managed." This quote, often attributed to management guru Peter Drucker, gets tossed around whenever the subject of stats and reporting comes up in business. Like it or not, without measurement, progress toward a goal is not possible. I want you to get excited about seeing the results. The numbers don't lie, and when you know how to interpret the reports, they guide your actions and decisions. As you'll discover in this chapter, tracking the activity in a practice can be simple and effective. When reviewed consistently, the reports will keep you responding proactively at the moment to the zigs and zags in your business. You'll be constantly investigating, tweaking, and adjusting your course so that hitting your target becomes inevitable. Even better, your COO can handle this and simply report what is being done to stay on course with the goals you set together.

Spreadsheets, Are They In or Out?

Let's just say spreadsheets are a thing of the past. While they may be a good option to use in other areas to track progress, I would argue that there are still better options you can use instead of spreadsheets. Needless to say, I'm not a big fan. Especially when you're trying to measure and report all of your business operations. Why would you when there are so many smart and savvy business intelligent (BI) systems you could use instead?!

What About PowerBI?

PowerBI is a great option as it has a reliable interface that will allow you to access a consolidated dashboard and pull reports on various analytics, enabling you to measure them efficiently. It's a solid choice, and many practices I work with currently use PowerBI to measure and track their growth. However, since I'm writing this book to give tips on efficiently maximizing your time and effort through simplification, I'm going to introduce you to another system that takes it one step further for orthodontists. So, for all your reporting and measuring business needs, let's talk about Gaidge.

Gaidge: The One-Stop-Shop for All Things Analytics

Gaidge is truly different from other systems because it's created solely for the orthodontic profession. Their mission is to "*simplify the business of orthodontics by providing easy-to-use practice metrics and business insights that efficiently report the health and progress of the practice, increasing business acumen and enhancing productivity and satisfaction for doctors and teams.".*

I spoke to Janet from AllSmiles about Gaidge since she is one of the handfuls of COOs currently using it to report and measure growth in their practice. She gave me a full rundown on how to use the system, why it's helpful, and why other practices should consider switching to Gaidge if they truly want to understand their progress and determine if they're meeting their goals.

What led AllSmiles to use Gaidge?

"We just liked that it was made specifically for orthodontists. It makes things so much easier because it's streamlined to our business goals. It's always about finding the right tools that work for you when it comes to your software systems. I'm sure there are others out there that help pull in your data, but before Gaidge, we would have to figure it out manually. Now, everything is so simple. You know how you're doing, and it's something you can look at every day at just a glance, just by looking at the dashboard."

Tell me about the Gaidge dashboard. What exactly am I looking at here?

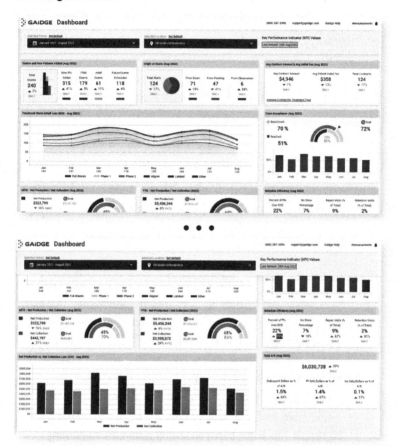

"That quick data is on the dashboard. If you look at the top right tab, you'll be able to input the start and end date of what you'd like to track, including your year-to-date, month-to-month, quarterly, or calendar year. There are numerous widgets on the page: 'Exams and New Patients Added,' 'Origin of Starts,' 'Average Contract Amount and Initial Fee,' 'Treatment Starts Detail,' and 'Case Acceptance.' You can also see your 'Month-to-Date

(MTD) and Year-to-Date (YTD) - Net Production/Net Collection,' 'Net Production vs. Net Collection,' 'Schedule Efficiency,' and 'Total A/R.' You can see all of these widgets at a glance, or you can click each of them to learn more. We must constantly monitor, measure, and analyze these things so we can stay on top of our goals and grow the practice to the targets we've created. You'll see we have goals and benchmarks for each of them, so I have to hold myself accountable and ensure we're doing what we can daily to reach them."

When you look at Gaidge at a glance, how do you know if everything is good or if you need to do something?

You can track all of your business goals on Gaidge. There's a function where you can manually write them in if you go to the settings. So, if you look at all of the widgets on the page, you'll notice that most have a benchmark or goal that I mentioned earlier. These are based on those goals you've entered. Each widget where it applies will show you what the goal is, your current percentage in reaching that goal, and if you're under or over the benchmark.

Is there a specific order to read this? For example, if I were to look at the 'Exams and New Patients Added' widget and see that the number of starts is below the benchmark, would I then look at the 'Origin of Starts' widget and see where to dive deeper and find out why?

"Yeah, you can do that. You can see where the drop happened by looking at 'Case Acceptance.' If you notice a particular month is down, you can find out why. That's a more involved process. I would have to see each

treatment coordinator's New Patient Tracker so we can gauge their performance to determine how many exams they've done, how many of those exams are starting, how many of them are going into 'Pending,' and how many of them are going into 'Observation/Recall.' For the ones going into 'Observation/Recall,' we don't have control over that since they're just not ready to start treatment due to their oral health, age, or other factors.

If I've determined the numbers for all those, I can go back to my 'Origin of Starts' and understand why some numbers are down. My 'Pending' list could be healthy, but my 'Observation/Recall' list could be high, and that's what's bringing that number down. All you can do in those cases is ensure your treatment coordinator always follows up and maintains that our practice will be there for them when they are ready to start treatment. They should send multiple reactivation campaigns to remember us as their primary orthodontist when they're ready."

How do you come up with these goals, and how frequently do they change?

"We set the goals usually once a year. We have a yearly planning meeting, but we meet bi-weekly to talk about where we're at, what we're doing, and how we can improve. We try to be proactive versus reactive when it comes to looking at things, so when I view the dashboard, I'll check to see if anything catches my attention that would trigger me to have a conversation with someone to ensure we're improving or not missing a step. Essentially, the goals help you stay accountable and take action when necessary. That's why it's great to have a system that concisely showcases everything."

Do you feel like you're reacting to things as they happen instead of seeing things after the fact when it's too late?

"For sure. I think it keeps you up-to-date instead of waiting until the end of the quarter to review your numbers. You can take action by observing the numbers in real-time, determining if you're trending downward, and asking the right questions to resolve the problem or at least understand why it's happening. It's better than looking back and thinking about all the ways you could have, should have, or would have fixed the problem. I recommend reviewing the dashboard weekly, so you don't fall too far behind or see trends and changes you don't want to see."

Do you use Gaidge in conjunction with PracticeBeacon to help you stay on track?

"Yeah, actually, I will use PracticeBeacon if I'm trying to understand the 'why' when analyzing the numbers in Gaidge. For example, if you look at the first widget, you'll see a total of 240 exams, and 315 new patients added. On my end, I would want to know why those other 85 people did not do an exam. Are they no-showing? Are they canceling? If they are, why is that happening? How did the scheduling coordinator do on the phone? Did they follow up with them? Is it something that we did that caused them not to come? To figure everything out, you can go to PracticeBeacon and listen to their new patient phone calls since they're recorded. Then, based on what I hear, I can coach and train from there to hopefully bring those numbers up."

With this system, you don't have to pull reports, right? Is there a time when you do have to pull reports?

"Right, because this system is automated, we don't have to pull reports. Everything stays up-to-date. However, if the starts from 'Observation/Recall' is down, we'll pull that report to ensure we can eventually get those people scheduled to start."

If you see that the number of new-patient starts is low, what do you do to try to increase those numbers?

"I think we're always looking at ways to market our practice. We can take on more new patients, whether the number is up or down. We always look for opportunities to do more community outreach, like sponsoring schools or sports teams and attending community events. I think we're covered well with help as far as digital marketing. Another way we bring those numbers up is by incentivizing our team. We'll create a goal that whoever gets a certain number of new patients this month will get a $100 gift card, for example. Many people are driven by money, so they're more likely to perform well when there's an incentive involved. We see a difference every time we do that, so it goes a long way."

Do you have any final insights you can provide on how to stay on top of tracking and make sure you're trending in the right direction?

"You should check in with the system a couple of times a week, discuss the results with your orthodontist, and address the problems as soon as possible. It helps to know who you should be speaking to for answers when you do need to resolve those issues quickly. So, for example, if

I'm trying to understand the exams and new patients, I will seek answers from the Patient Care Centre. Or, if I'm determining what's going on with the 'Origin of Starts' and 'Case Acceptance,' or even something like the 'Average Patient Initial Fee,' I'll want to pull in the treatment coordinator for answers. It's a collaborative effort. We all want to see growth and progress, and we're all doing our best to make that happen. So, it's best to stay on top and avoid letting any details fall through the cracks."

If you'd like to learn more about Gaidge, scan these QR codes to watch an interview about tracking and reporting and request a free demo!

Add QR code here:

Gaidge is the best reporting software for orthodontists, in my opinion, because it provides the exact functionality necessary to stay on top of an orthodontic practice. Other business intelligence systems like Power BI are so robust that they can be overwhelming.

At this point, all the pieces are in place for rapid growth. As growth continues, you'll reach a stage where you are maximizing the output of your current location and wondering about the next steps to sustain your growth rate. When is the right time to open a satellite office, and how do you do it effectively? In Chapter 7, we'll discuss what you need to know about opening another location.

CHAPTER 7

Scaling Your Practice with Satellite Locations

We're almost at the final stretch, and so far, you're equipped to take these tools and make some magic. If you think about it, it's been a long journey together. Over the last three books, you've learned how to create the front desk of your dreams, cultivate the ultimate treatment coordinator, and recently, scale your practice by perfecting your operations. Many chapters, processes, procedures, cases, and words of wisdom later, you now know how to create a scalable practice successfully. Whether your goal is to grow into a medium- or large-sized practice, you can now start by feeling confident that you have the proper tools and resources to guide you through it.

To do this right the first time around, you have to ensure that you have:

- A vision for your practice.

- An integrator to implement that vision.

- The right org chart that has the right people in the right seats.

- A strong brand and culture.

- An exceptional hiring and onboarding process.

- Top-notch systems to measure and report your growth.

It would be best if you executed each of those things to its full potential and capacity to see exponential growth. And the most important part? Consistency, because true growth only occurs when true consistency is maintained. Once you've successfully mastered all these things in your practice, you can now think about replicating the process in another location and opening up a satellite. But before you run to secure a lease on a building, let's first go over what you should consider before you open up a satellite practice.

The Satellite Practice: Case Study

Case 1: Dr. Johnson

Two years ago, Dr. Johnson took over a small practice in his hometown in Denver, Colorado. Being the only orthodontist in town, it was quite an easy transition as his new office was close to a middle school, so the demand for new patients was constant. Dr. Johnson kept all the previous staff on his team, including the moody front desk coordinator, Alice, even though she always rolled her eyes when the phone rang and called in sick at least once per week. Not only that, but she continuously missed calls and often did not return prospective patients' calls. But still, Dr. Johnson felt bad as she had been there five years with the previous doctor, so he kept her on. After all, the business was doing fine. His treatment coordinator, Mona, saw about four to five prospective patients per day and usually ran her exams for an hour. She wanted to take on more patients, but she also worked as Dr. Johnson's clinical assistant during her shifts, which made it difficult to book new patients for consultations. He manually inputted all operational matters on a spreadsheet that needed to be updated frequently.

This continued for about ten months until Dr. Johnson noticed that his production numbers had stagnated, and the practice was no longer growing and had reached a plateau. The only marketing he ever did was pay for an ad in the local newspaper. But he had an idea. He believed that if he opened up a second practice, he'd make more money. Six months later, he decided to open a satellite a few towns over, as there, again, was no competition and the lease was cheap. He had his staff work part-time at the primary practice and part-time at his satellite. He even re-designed his ad to include both of his locations. But a few months in, Dr. Johnson began to regret his decision. Not only was he getting complaints about poor customer service in both locations, but he also noticed that his treatment coordinator was only getting about 1-2 patients per day for consultations. He also started to regret his design decisions, as his satellite looked very different from his original location. Most people didn't even realize the same person owned them. Eight months later, Dr. Johnson closed his satellite, fired his front desk coordinator, and decided to focus on building his primary practice up again. He knew he had done things wrong and needed to make a change.

Case 2: Dr. Smith

Four years ago, Dr. Smith began his mission to turn his small boutique office into a large scalable practice within ten years. He envisioned opening eight practices in and outside the city of Sacramento, California, and wanted to bring in eight figures in production annually. To do this successfully, Dr. Smith knew he needed to put all his thoughts on paper, so he used the Operating System to help get him started. He wanted to do things the right way the first time, so he included his team in his vision from the get-go and had them buy into it. He implemented a few things, such as an automated CRM system for lead generation, external and digital marketing to increase his exposure, and the proper process for hiring and onboarding to attract the right talent. He even hired more people than necessary to ensure he had all hands on deck to take on more new patients and keep the practice in ship shape. He always incentivized the hard work of his team with gift cards, bonuses, and contests.

After two years, Dr. Smith went from doing $500,000 to $3,000,000 in production. As he encountered new growth, he continued to hire and update his processes to ensure everyone remained on the same page. He also realized that he was no longer able to do it on his own, so he hired a COO, Kevin, to run the day-to-day while he focused on patient care. Dr. Smith was happy with the way his practice was running, however, after realizing that his staff were working to their full capacity and were unable to fit new patients into their schedule, he decided it was time to open a second location. The satellite was 20 minutes away from the practice, but Dr. Smith made sure it was in a location nearby dozens of subdivisions, multiple schools, and a busy commercial area.

He hired a new group of people who were trained by the original team to ensure they followed the same processes and procedures and brought on another doctor, Dr. Minh, to help out with patient care. Dr. Smith was consistent throughout his growth, and he now has four satellites in booming locations and 40 happy employees. He's six years from his 10-year goal, with four practices to go and a large potential of money to be made.

Case Analysis

Dr. Johnson could look at his experience in hindsight and acknowledge the reasons why the success of his practice began to dwindle and what ultimately led to the closure of his first satellite. He'd probably come to understand that:

- His customer service was terrible.

- He kept an onboard terrorist on staff.

- His treatment coordinator's exams were too long.

- His staff was not following the right processes and procedures.

- He didn't have a CRM system (I.e., PracticeBeacon).

- He should not have had Mona do both the treatment coordinator role and the clinical assistant role.

- He opened up a new satellite without addressing the issues in his primary practice.

- He opened up a new satellite in the wrong location.

- He didn't spend money on marketing.

- He ran the business and provided patient care.

Whereas Dr. Smith could acknowledge that the success of his practices comes from various things, like:

- He had buy-in from his team.
- He had a vision.
- He documented a 10-year plan.
- He automated his systems.
- He increased his internal and external marketing.
- He hired the right people to fill the right seats.
- He staffed more than he needed.
- He incentivized his staff.
- He updated his processes every time a change occurred.
- He hired a COO so he could focus on being an orthodontist.
- He opened his first satellite when he perfected his model and was at full capacity.
- He opened the satellite in the right location.
- He kept training consistently.
- He kept his brand and culture consistent.
- He brought another doctor on board to help with patient care.

Effectively Maintaining a Satellite

So, if you've learned anything from Dr. Johnson and Dr. Smith's cases, you'll realize the four main things you'll need to effectively maintain a satellite: a model that works, a schedule at full capacity, the proper location, and the ability to predict future hot spots.

The Bullet-Proof Model

Having a model that's been tried and tested is crucial to the success and growth of your practice. Everything has to be perfected before you decide to replicate it, or you'll be dealing with the same issues in both practices. That means you must have:

- The right people to fill the right seats.
- Effective training and coaching methods.
- A strong leadership team.
- A positive brand and culture.
- Efficient systems.

When each of these things is effective and reliable, you'll have the confidence to repeat the same process in your satellite. This is who you are. This is how you'll continue to be known.

The Maximized Schedule

Before you even think about opening up a satellite, your first thought should always be about how you can maximize your current location and schedule. You've put your heart and soul into opening up your practice, so why not allow your primary practice to reach its full potential before branching out? You'll want to consider how many prospective patients you could bring on before you reach full capacity. If you're comfortable with the size of your practice, you probably have that capped at a number that you don't plan on surpassing at the location you're currently at. That's the number of spots your front desk coordinator can schedule without being overbooked. That's the number your treatment coordinators can fit into one day while ensuring each exam is 30 minutes or less and they take their necessary breaks. If you've hit that number, then consider opening up a second location for new patients to visit.

Location, Location, Location

If you've watched any real estate shows on HGTV, you've probably heard every agent in every episode say the cliché phrase, "location, location, location." It's not just important to consider when buying a house. Opening a practice in the right location is also paramount to its success. This ultimately looks different for everybody, but you shouldn't expect dramatic growth if you're opening up a practice in a remote area with a small population away from neighborhoods and schools (Obviously, but always important to point out blatantly). Instead, look for locations that are in or near other commercial spaces, close to schools, and in neighborhoods with young families, especially those lacking orthodontic services.

Hot-Spot Predictions

Pay attention to up-and-coming areas in your community to determine where and when to open up your satellite practice. New developments are constantly arising as the population grows, and you can usually tell which towns are at the beginning of their boom. Keep those places in mind and keep track of their progress. If you start to notice new housing developments, schools, churches, and commercial spaces being sold, you'll want to keep a space in that area on your radar.

I remember one call I made to Dr. Fishbein about opening up a satellite in this community outside of Pensacola when they were in their early stages of development. Dr. Fishbein noticed they were near completion in two of the schools they were building, so he called me to discuss my suggestion more. "Hey, I'm driving around the area that you mentioned. Where should I open an office?" he asked. "You need to open it very close to Nine Mile Road and Pine Forest Road, somewhere within a mile or two of that area," I advised him. He ended up opening this satellite a mile down the street, right on Nine Mile Road, in a brand new complex, right next to the dental clinic of one of his friends (who opened it simultaneously). As a result, they now have a referral network, and the Cantonment location ended up being Dr. Fishbein's fastest-growing satellite.

Now, providing clients with advice on where to open their practice isn't one of the services I offer. It happened after developing a friendship with Dr. Fishbein, and it helped that we live in the same town. However, some people specialize in startups. They can analyze the markets and provide insights on the best locations to open up your new business. You should research that, but in the meantime, you could check out Choosing the Right Practice Location by Jayme Amos on how to choose the right practice location. It's written for dental practices, but the same rules apply!

Best Practices to Consider

Now that you know how to do things the right way, we can get started on what this process looks like. The first thing to determine is how much you need to be producing in a duration of time to even open a satellite. Dr. Fishbein got it down to a formula where he could open a new satellite by producing $2,000,000 in 24 months. So, it's important to understand your budget and work with your accountant to help you understand your timeline without going into massive debt. Once that's all taken care of, and your ideal location has been found, you can dive right into setting up your satellite. If you want to stay true to your brand and culture, you should just be doing exactly what you did the first time around! That means replicating your design, staffing the right people, and using the same operating system.

There are a few tips you may want to consider when you open your first satellite. This advice will help you do things right the first time so you can save yourself trouble in the future:

1. **Open each location part-time to start and get your team to travel between them.**

   Most orthodontists who open their first satellite will get their team to split their time between both locations on a part-time basis. They'll be able to get the satellite up and running, so the transition pains are a little less stressful, as the team is already fully trained and well-versed in the operating systems and processes you have in place. They may spend time there once or twice a week, while the rest of their time is spent in the primary practice. As things settle and the satellite begins to scale, you can eventually hire a new team that solely works in the satellite. I know many orthodontists who currently do this, as their satellites are within the same community. But as you continue to grow and open up more satellites, getting your team to travel between them doesn't end up working so well. You have to go into it as a temporary practice, and your goal should always be to maximize each location with a designated team and a full schedule of patients.

2. Plan to hire an associate doctor, either on a salary or per diem basis.

If you desire to grow your practice so you can have more hands on deck to spend more personal time doing the things you love, you may not want to travel between both locations and work so much. If that's the case, it might be wise to hire another doctor to help take on the new set of patients this new location will provide. This could be a salary position where they're working a set amount of days per week, or it could also be on a per diem basis if you're not fully sold on the idea of getting a new doctor on salary right away. I know a few orthodontists who have taken this route to help with their multiple locations. These doctors aren't on staff, but they have contracts to fill in one or two days per week. This will allow you to test things out first without paying a big salary—you just pay them on the days they come in.

3. Don't open satellites you don't plan on using.

I've met a few orthodontists who open satellites they don't use. There's absolutely no sense in opening nine different locations but only using four of them to capacity. I even know a few orthodontists who have locations they use maybe once or twice per month. In these cases, you end up developing a list of regular patients in each of those locations, and before you know it, six months roll by, and you start to realize that you can't fit in any more new patients because your schedule is full. This, in my opinion, is a waste of time, money, and resources. If you don't hire more staff and open more days throughout the week (or month), those satellites will always be at a standstill. So, the rule of thumb here is if you can't maximize the location and grow into it, then you don't need to open it. If you can't open a location and immediately be there at least one day per week, it's best to let that location go. It's best practice to start at one day and add more from there, depending on how much you and your team can handle.

4. Try to maximize your satellites within two years.

Your goal should be to have each satellite working at full capacity, and two years should be an ample amount of time to get you there. That means following the advice I provided in points 1, 2, and 3 so that you can make that goal a reality. Just like you shouldn't open a satellite if your primary practice isn't fully maximized, the same goes for your satellites. Every location has to be top-notch before you even consider moving further. So, work with your COO, your leadership team, and your accountants. Make sure everyone involved has full confidence in moving forward. If they don't and there are still a few gaps that need to be filled, take your time to do that efficiently to ensure you're taking the proper action to eventually meet your goals.

When I spoke to Dr. Despot about the growth of his practice, I wanted to know what his thought process was when he was getting his first satellite up and running. Dr. Despot, like many others, knew how important it was to maximize his first location before he even thought about the venture.

Dr. Despot, how did you decide it was the right time to open a second location?

> *"I felt like we were at full capacity at our first location. Things were starting to plateau. The previous year, we had grown 58%, and we knew we couldn't reach anywhere close to that number in the future. We could see some trends showing us that future growth would not happen. So, we just decided that it was the right time to do it, and we had the right amount of cash to make it happen seamlessly."*

How did you decide on where that second location would be?

> *"I'm in Texas, and the market is growing quickly here. There are some cities over here that are just exploding, so we looked at the second fastest-growing city in Texas, which is Leander. We said that's where we want to be, and we must get there before somebody else. It was just a really attractive spot. Part of our demographics in finding a spot is that we want to be across the street from the middle school because that's our patient base. Our*

target market is the moms of middle schoolers. But our patient base is middle schoolers, making it convenient for their moms. We got ourselves a spot right across the street from a middle school with well over 1000 kids in it. Every year there are new kids, new kids, new kids, which means new patients, new patients, new patients."

You sound like you have the right operating systems in place for that to happen. Would you say you and your team have perfected them?

"Yes, but our operating systems are always changing in that we always want to improve and get better. We're always looking for ways to stay on top and tweak as needed. You have to. The world is changing so quickly. Look at what happened to poor BlockBuster because they didn't make any changes. We have a lot of really cool systems in place, but at the top corner of each page of our system, it has the date when it was last updated, and we're frequently updating them. We're trying new things to see how each of them works for a little while and figure out a way to measure it, so we know if it's a successful change or not. We can always revert if it doesn't work. We have to ensure they're being updated in each location to keep things consistent, so the communication has to be there for everyone to understand where we're currently at."

What advice would you give to people looking to open a second location?

"Consistency is key. You know, there's a reason that folks get a burger at McDonald's. It's because they know what they'll get every single time. That's what we want. We

want to have the same thing every single time in both of our locations. We want patients to have the same positive experience. We want them to feel the same way when they leave each one of our locations. We want them to feel like they're leaving in a better mood than they came in. You have to have systems in place for that and duplicate that in every location that you own, and ensure your team is always executing everything you've set out consistently."

Do You Feel Ready to Move Forward?

If you're feeling confident about moving forward in this growth process and are excited about scaling your practice, then I'm happy to say you're in the right frame of mind to get this ball rolling! We're now at the point in our growth series where we can put it all together and give you an overview of what your mindset has to be to get you to successfully get through these next steps. In the next and final chapter, we'll re-evaluate your "why" and reveal the best practices you should consider to ensure you're in the right mindset to get you to your desired goals.

8

Planning Your Next Steps With A Growth Mindset

As you plan your next steps and implement everything you've learned, it's important to come full circle and revisit the reason that brought you here: a desire to grow your practice.

Currently, the average orthodontic practice produces 1.2 million dollars a year. Before rising inflation costs over the last two decades, 80% of orthodontists coming out of residency started their own practice, while the other 20% became associates. Today, those numbers are reversed. It has become increasingly difficult to be a business owner due to the rising cost of living. When you look at how much you spent on dental school and residency alone, 1.2 million in production doesn't leave you much to take home and pay off your debts.

That's why I wanted to create this book series in the first place. I want to show new doctors—who have taken on the challenge of opening a practice—how to take the right steps from the beginning so they don't get on the hamster wheel. For experienced doctors whose practices' may have plateaued a while ago, I want to show them the changes they must make to their current structure to break through, start growing again, and rekindle their passion. By just making over the national average of 1.2 million, you will be in the top 2 to 3% of all orthodontic practices. These people are doing things differently, things that most orthodontists never do. So, you can be a 3, 5, 10, or 20 million-dollar practice; it doesn't matter to me. It's about you and your goal and what you must do to rise above average. That can only happen when implementing a growth mindset.

Deciding What You Want

Deciding what you want comes down to these two questions: Do you want a lifestyle practice or a scalable practice? Are you in it for the money or the mission? After reading the last seven chapters (and if you've had a chance to read them, *Front Desk Secrets and The Ultimate Treatment Coordinator*), you may finally know how to answer those two questions.

If you've felt uneasy about making these changes to your current practice and feel more comfortable working with a small team and making a decent living, you probably want to remain a lifestyle practice. That's not a bad thing! You want to fill your schedule, put food on your table, pay your staff, and be an orthodontist and business owner. 90% of orthodontists run practices like this. If you feel this way, I hope you can still take some insights I've shared and apply them to your practice. You should still want a positive work culture, effective processes and systems, and happy staff members to provide the best services possible for your patients. This alone can do wonders for a smaller lifestyle practice.

However, if reading these books has piqued your interest and left you hungry to learn more, you've probably already been thinking about what type of mission you need to be on to scale your practice and have a clear vision in place. Be honest about what you want and how long you think it will take you to get there. Growth looks different for everyone.

If you have a goal to achieve an annual production of $5,000,000 in one location in five years, maybe that means adopting the medium-sized org chart, hiring more specialized roles, and implementing efficient CRM and BI systems, like PracticeBeacon and Gaidge, to support all your operational needs. If you're happy with that number and know it's enough, go for it and make it happen. But if you have a goal to achieve an annual production of $20,000,000, you'll need a more complex structure that involves more doctors and a longer time frame. More time, effort, resources, processes, staff, and planning will have to go into this to ensure you can fulfill your mission. A plan of this nature requires investment, so you must be okay with taking that money right off your bottom line to bring your vision to life. You have to hire a COO to integrate your vision, and you have to be okay with paying them a six-figure salary.

It's just about deciding what will make you happy. You don't have to be that 20-million-dollar practice. It might sound appealing, for sure, but it's not worth it if the journey itself won't make you happy. We are working with a practice that has just reached the 5-million-dollar mark, and they're comfortable staying at that level. The CEO has an associate and two locations. He probably takes home around 1.5 million, spends a lot of time with his family, and takes many great vacations. He knows he and his team still have to be somewhat aggressive with the marketing and events he does in his community to maintain a great reputation, but he's throttling it to keep it around its current size. What matters is you take the appropriate steps to let change happen so that you and your staff can be satisfied.

Making the Proper Investments

A few months ago, I spoke with an orthodontist interested in learning more about HIP's services. He's been in practice for over 25 years and has a small practice that brings in just over a million dollars. I could tell he was frustrated with the lack of growth his practice has experienced over the years, and overall didn't seem happy. He wanted to make changes, but when I began to discuss the types of things he could do to grow, he complained about everything being too expensive. The conversation ended with him asking how he could shave off every penny possible to take more home at the end of the day. With this mindset, he'll never go anywhere. He will remain at this level of production for another 25 years.

You need to spend money to make money. That's just how it works. Just ask Richard Branson or Elon Musk if they penny-pinched when they created Virgin or Tesla. I'll tell you one thing: you would have never heard about these billion-dollar companies if they did.

"A penny saved is a penny earned." While this is a good proverb to live by in everyday life, it doesn't serve you when trying to grow a business. You can save up a thousand pennies, but it will be worth nothing if you don't invest it. It should be invested in the things that bring you cash flow. When my company, HIP, does external, digital marketing for a practice, they are marketing to a brand new audience who can become new patient consultations. If you hire more people to grow your team, you have more staff who can turn these new patients into starts. More starts mean more production. More production means more investment capital for growth. Ultimately, if you can create cash flow that outpaces the debt and interest on the debt, why wouldn't you do that?

Don't be complacent or comfortable with where you are, and avoid doing more because you're afraid of what it will cost you. This is a trap people get stuck in without ever realizing their potential. Don't think about what your org chart is costing you. The value in your patient experience far outweighs the cost of your org chart. If your people create the best experience for your patients, you will generate the cash flow on the back end. Spending your time fearing the additional costs means you and your team are doing more work, leaving all involved burnt out, frustrated, and resentful. Ultimately, it comes down to taking a risk and a giant leap of faith. But I promise, by the end of it, you'll be surprised when you realize you've exceeded what you thought was even possible.

Laying Out a Plan

Everyone's plan will look different. Take Dr. Fishbein, for example. He knew he wanted to grow his practice, but it would take a lot of time and effort since he didn't have the cash right away. He knew he wanted to promote his then-treatment coordinator, Amanda, to a managerial position, but he did it in phases. He promised her that if the practice grew, she would keep getting bumps in her salary and job title changes. He laid a plan for her, and she bought into it and went along for the ride.

"I just told her, 'When we get to this phase, you'll get this money and this title. When we get to that phase, you'll get that amount and that title. I laid it all out for her from the start for her to see so she knew I was serious. And

she held me accountable for it. Eventually, we made a plan for her to become the COO where she was running the show, and I was seeing the patients."

Dr. Fishbein luckily had Amanda from the start. She's been with him over the last decade. For others, that's not always the case. Since you're just starting your growth journey, I would advise you to find the right people, be transparent about what growth looks like, and get them to buy into your vision so they can feel confident in growing with you. You never know if one of them will eventually be COO material. If that's not the case, you'll have taken the necessary steps, set up the right systems, and made the investments that create the cash flow you need to hire a COO without sweating the six-figure salary.

Creating the Right Culture

When I think about the average practices currently bringing in around 1.2 million (or less), there's usually one thing they all have in common: a non-existent culture. I've stepped into a few of these practices, where I've just been surrounded by white walls, a row of chairs, and a glass window separating reception from the rest of the room. Most of the time, you're greeted by Roz from Monsters, Inc., who's usually annoyed when she says, "Can I help you?" There's no "Hi, how are you?" Nothing. It's bleak.

If your office currently looks like this, I'm not trying to offend you. I'm just telling you the truth and hinting that you need to be making changes right now. Paint your walls, remove your glass barriers, and make your office a place for people to enjoy. Build a team that is fun, bubbly, hard-working, social, and driven. Get that Roz character away from the phones and front desk!! (Newsflash—she's an onboard terrorist). You have to create that positive, uplifting energy, and you have to think of all of the ways you can make that happen. To improve the culture in your practice, you can start by asking yourself simple questions like:

- What are my core values?
- Do my people share the same core values?
- How do I want people to feel when they enter my practice?
- How do I make sure my staff always have a positive attitude while they're working?
- Am I hiring people who want to provide the best patient experience?
- How can I make people feel more comfortable when they come to my practice?
- Does my office feel inviting?
- Am I doing things that make people motivated to work?
- Do I celebrate wins or just penalize faults?

By reflecting on these questions first, you'll be able to acknowledge areas that need improvement and take the right course of action to do so. For example, if you want your staff and patients to feel more comfortable and at ease, consider ditching the standard waiting room chairs and adding a few couches. If you want your office to be more inviting, try painting your walls a bright color and putting up a photo wall of your staff and patients. If you find yourself constantly dishing negative feedback, celebrate them when they do something great. If you need your staff to work together better, there are countless team-building exercises you can try to improve morale, boost collaboration, and increase satisfaction in your team. And if you need help envisioning all of this, visit and speak with other practices for inspiration! This boost in your culture is only going to better your brand!

Dr. Fishbein didn't just wake up one morning and magically know what to do to improve his practice. He knew he needed help to change his mindset, so he learned from the big dogs before him to help lay his foundation.

> *"When I first started, I had no idea. You have to unlearn everything you learned in school to get out of the orthodontist mindset and into the business mindset. That's hard to do when you're still trying to be a good orthodontist. I learned very quickly that I couldn't do both. I sucked at being a business owner, and I knew I needed help. So, when I was first trying to get things going, I would visit the biggest practices near me, literally anyone I could find who would let me visit and see what*

their mindset was and determine what they were doing that was successful. I learned from the big dogs at that time."

Dr. Farina has a long list of core values that he showcases on the wall of his hallway for all to see as they pass by. He loves to get his team pumped and encourages them to have fun while working, and you can see each of their personalities shine when you walk in. They know the goal, and they are excited to meet that goal every day. It also helps that they have an awesome building to work in, far from the visuals of your standard medical facility. All these things combined create Dr. Farina's fantastic culture that he has worked so hard to achieve. At this point, it's paid off. With these changes, Dr. Farina has almost doubled his annual production in the two years since we started working with him. He and his team are well on their way to producing more.

Want to learn more? Scan here to learn more about Dr. Farina and how he sets his practice apart from the competition through his culture.

Developing a Growth Mindset

Simply making these small changes will create drastic changes in your practice's culture. It all comes down to your vision and implementing the tactical elements to create it, like nailing your core values and DNA and having a growth mindset. You're going to want to develop those things. You can't just say, "We're just here to put braces on teeth," and expect to scale. You have to be in the right mindset to improve your culture to promote your brand. For this to happen, you have to have the right energy. Energy is contagious. When it comes from you first, it will transfer to everyone else in your practice. And soon enough, you'll all be operating with the same energy.

Many of the practices I work with swear by the team huddle. They say it's the best way to start the workday with your team to get everyone pumped and excited to work. They do this every single morning before they start working. I recommend doing this with your own team. They might feel awkward about it initially, but I promise you, if you approach it with the right energy, they will buy in. You can start your huddle by asking your staff if they have a "win" they'd like to share with the team. It can be as simple as, "I went to the beach yesterday on my day off," or "Sally got her braces off, and her smile was perfect. She cried and said coming to our practice has changed her life." Just starting your morning huddle with a few wins will help everyone get into the right mindset for the remainder of the day. It's really that simple.

As the CEO, you're responsible for deciding what your brand and culture look like, which must be reflected throughout your practice. You, along with your leadership team, have to keep your team on the right path so they are constantly maintaining your vision. You have a responsibility to protect that and ensure there aren't any onboard terrorists around to destroy it. So, what can you do to ensure you and your leadership team are putting in the effort to maintain positive energy to ignite your brand and culture?

Let's Get Energized!

There are many activities you can do together with your leadership team, but one that I particularly like is creating a book club. You can take turns selecting a book about leadership and share one thing you've learned from that book during your team meetings. If you have a team Slack channel or Facebook group, you can drop a quote on the page whenever something inspires you.

We do this with our team at HIP, ensuring prospective candidates know all about it in the hiring process. Why? Because it's not for everyone. Some people just want to work at a job to receive a paycheck. They don't like the team-building exercises or the motivational channel we live by because it makes them uncomfortable. And honestly, we've had people leave HIP for these exact reasons. Now we've learned to bring it up early on in the interview process, as it lets us know if they're interested in joining that type of environment. This ensures that the culture at HIP is always maintained, protected, and respected by each member of my team.

Another way to foster positive energy (and probably the most critical) is by investing in yourself. We get caught up in the trials and tribulations of life once in a while. It can be overwhelming to manage work life, family life, and social life while also trying to have a bit of 'you' time. Sometimes, it's quite hard to put ourselves first. But here's what happens when you don't: you end up taking on more and more and more without taking the time to digest it all, and eventually, you'll just burn out. So, focus on what makes you happy in your downtime.

I implement my Morning Formula every single day, as that's what puts me in the right mind frame to start my day off right. Then, I'll listen to an audiobook on my way to work. Investing in oneself looks different for everyone. It could be going on vacation for a few days, planning a golf day with your friends, getting your hair and nails done at the salon, or working out every morning.

You have to take the time and space to practice self-care, or else you will find your energy will dwindle more and more every passing day.

And what's a Morning Formula, you ask? Scan here to learn about it.

Dr. Despot and Janet Moser know the importance of self-care to maintain the proper mindset to be the CEO and COO of each of their practices.

Dr. Despot says:

> *"You've got to take clarity breaks whenever you can, even if you leave the office and get lost in your thoughts when you have a few moments to spare. Sometimes, it's necessary to walk away from something you're working on, do something that will ease your mind, and approach it later with a fresh set of eyes."*

Janet believes:

> *"I think it's important to ensure that you take care of yourself first above everything else. Once you do that, you're better able to show up for others and be the best version of yourself for them. My version of self-care used to be the gym, but that became difficult to continue after having my first baby. So now I've changed things up a bit, and I'm practicing self-care from home. I will often meditate and use my Peloton as much as I can. It's not always easy, but it's necessary."*

One final thing I will suggest is for you and your COO to read The New One-Minute Manager. The whole premise of this book is to praise or correct action within one minute so people receive immediate feedback. Whether they make a mistake or do something amazing, you should be able to either correct or praise the action or behavior concisely. This is a great approach to take as your people will understand right then and there if they are operating out of the integrity of the culture of the practice. You can't have your COO waiting for quarterly reviews to give feedback or "sweeping things under the rug" when people are either not doing their part or being acknowledged for their hard work. The New One-Minute Manager is an audiobook you can listen to in under an hour. Scan here to purchase and give it a listen! [And eventually, send it to your future COO]. I promise it will change how you think about your management style, enabling you to provide effective feedback to your team.

Planning Your Next Steps

If reading this has been like drinking from a fire hose and you're struggling with where to start, don't worry. Let's go over the steps you can take right now to get this process started.

Step 1: Download the Orthodontic Practice Operating System

This is where it all begins. Download the template, take a few days to think about each of the questions, book a meeting with your team, and discuss your goals for the practice. Go over each question and have a thoughtful discussion about everyone's feelings towards it. You'll know right then and there who is on board and who will probably not stay with you for this journey. Take the time to fill out the questions in a concise, clear manner and ensure that everyone agrees with each answer. In case you didn't download it earlier, now is the time to get serious and

SCAN ME

download it now. Here's the QR code again, so you don't have to frantically search for it.

Step 2: Contact Wiseman Strategies

Wiseman Strategies is the first company you'll want to get in touch with, as they'll help you plan out your org chart and find the right people to fill the right seats. Specifically, they will determine the different kinds of roles you'll need, discuss the vision for each of the roles, outline the compensation packages, and provide you with qualified candidates. You'll especially want to reach out to them to help you find your COO because, as I've reiterated countless times, you should NOT be running the operations of your practice any longer by yourself.

"What if I want to promote one of my staff members to the COO role?" you might ask. If you have a rockstar employee who you think might fit the COO criteria, definitely consider that! Your employees work hard, and they deserve growth opportunities. Fishbein and AllSmiles saw the potential in Amanda and Janet, both working in the COO role. If you'd like to go this route, Wiseman Strategies can provide you with a Predictive Index (PI) behavioral assessment that your employee can take to see if it aligns with the attributes of a COO and the responsibilities the role entails.

I've worked with Wiseman Strategies for a couple of years now, and I would not have the team I have today without their expertise and support. Give them a call! Scan this QR code to visit their website, where you can find their details and contact information. But before you do, listen to the full interview with the team at Wiseman Strategies.

Step 3: Contact HIP!

Once you've hired your new team members and expanded your departments, you'll want to make sure your team gets the proper training so they're fully able to provide the best patient care and utilize your systems. Then, you'll want to increase your internal and external marketing so your brand can shine to a new audience on various channels. This is where my team and I at HIP can help. We offer asynchronous and synchronous online training modules for your entire team, an all-in-one CRM system (PracticeBeacon) to help track your leads and manage your schedule, a complete website revamp, and digital marketing via all social media channels! We have helped hundreds of orthodontic practices build bigger practices and powerful brands to turn prospective patients into profits. If you want to learn more about who we are, what we offer, and how to get in contact, visit www.hip.agency.

Final Note

Writing this book has been the culmination of my life's work and purpose. What I've shared in these pages has come through my experience and values of personal growth, life-long learning, taking action, and serving others. While the first two books in the Orthodontic Practice Growth Series are essential to cultivation and acquisition, this book is the foundation for an orthodontic business. It's what you can use to overcome your growing pains, and it's the basis that all thriving practices use to build their success.

Throughout the whole journey, the key to success is mindset. The common denominator among all the top 1% orthodontic practices is the growth mindset. People with a growth mindset will always find a way to do great things regardless of their conditions. This has long been a passion of mine, and it is the subject of the last book in this series. Stay tuned for its release at the end of 2022.

It has been my privilege to serve in this profession for the past eight years. I have learned so much from the amazing doctors I have met.

I look forward to serving you for years to come.

Best,

Luke Infinger

Made in USA - Kendallville, IN
97600_9781990476082
03.30.2024 1152